M.E. and My Ducks

To Christine

Best Wishes

all my love

Linda J. Howard.

M.E. and My Ducks

LINDA J. HOWARD

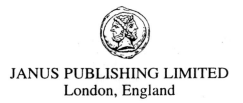

JANUS PUBLISHING LIMITED
London, England

First published in Great Britain 1996
by Janus Publishing Company
Edinburgh House, 19 Nassau Street
London W1N 7RE

British Library Cataloguing-in-Publication Data.
A catalogue record for this book is available from the British Library.

ISBN 1 85756 207 0

Cover design Harold King

Photosetting by Keyboard Services, Luton, Beds
Printed and bound in England by
Antony Rowe Ltd
Chippenham
Wiltshire

TO A WONDERFUL MAN

Oh Dad you were a wonderful man,
So kind, so brave, so strong,
Why did you leave us in such a rush?
To us it seemed so wrong.

There's Mum and Carol, Janet and me,
We have cried so many tears,
Since the day that you left us, it was so quick,
After so many wonderful years.

We know that you are now out of pain,
We wouldn't wish it different, darling Dad,
To see you asleep and Resting in Peace,
It is for us, that we feel so sad.

You will always be with us, this I know,
Your presence is with us today,
We shall talk to you daily, well I know I will,
God's told me you're not far away.

God bless you and keep you till we meet again.

Your Loving Daughter Linda.

Chapter One

I have always lived a very busy and full life, running the home, working part-time and raising two sons and two stepsons. My hobbies were gardening, cake-making, knitting, walking and bird-watching and in my spare time I would find something else to do. As long as I was busy, I was happy.

My husband, Vic, and I had spent twelve months renovating an old flat that had been neglected for many years. It was easy to work on it in the evenings and at weekends because we already had somewhere else to live. Vic was a caretaker of a

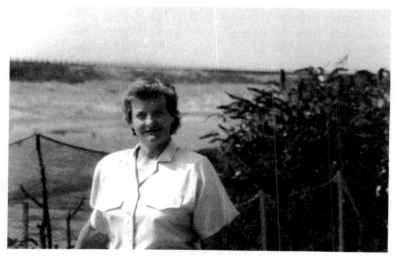

Linda in the garden overlooking Widewater.

very large school in Steyning and had been there for almost twenty years. We both felt we needed a change, so Vic was going to go back to his original trade as an electrician, and that meant we would have to find somewhere to live, because the house we were living in came with the job.

Our new home is in Lancing, West Sussex. It is an upstairs flat, but it is built on the side of a bank, so that the lower flat is on road level and our flat above is ground level to the back. So we also have a garden. But what is unique about the place is the lagoon at the bottom of the garden. It is about a mile long and thirty-three feet wide and is fed from the sea and rain water from the Downs, so it is saline water. On the opposite side of the lagoon is another bank which is a sea defence, because beyond that is the English Channel.

Living on the lagoon, which is called Widewater, were a pair of swans and just a few mallard ducks. We thought they were wonderful but we never realised how important they were going to be in my life in later years. When we first viewed the flat we realised that it needed a great deal of hard work and money spent on it. But that didn't matter as we had fallen in love with the place. It was so relaxing to just sit and listen to the water and see the wildlife – it was so very different from living on the school premises.

It wasn't until we had purchased the property and taken a good look round that we realised just what we had taken on. None of the windows fitted, the front door didn't close properly, there was no central heating and the kitchen just had a sink unit, a rotten draining board, and no fitted cupboards or hot water. We knew all this when we bought the place, but when it was empty of the other owner's belongings it made everything else look ten times worse. But this didn't seem to be a problem – we were both fit, healthy and eager to get on with it.

We would spend nearly every weekend working on the flat, pulling out old gas pipes, ripping up floor boards and replacing plumbing. You name it, we did it, and we really enjoyed every minute. The best part of the day was at dusk, when we would make ourselves a cup of coffee and go and sit on the grass and watch the pair of swans and half a dozen mallards preening themselves on the water. If it was a clear night the moon would shine down on the water and make it look so lovely. Sometimes

I would want the clocks to stop so that time would stand still for evermore. But that would never happen and we would have to pack up and go back to our house and reality. Until the next weekend.

The garden never got a look-in for the first few months – it was just used to store things or dump things as it was only grass and weeds and, anyway, it was a continuous slope, so you couldn't use it to sit in. In fact, that isn't quite true – if I put a towel on the grass and sat on it then dug my heels into the grass, I could have a well-earned cup of tea and watch the wildlife before my towel and I reached the water's edge. I started taking bread out to feed the ducks when we had our breaks and a neighbour said that they liked fresh water as the lagoon was too salty. So I gave them clean water every weekend and gradually the ducks and swans became very tame and they knew they would get bread and water fresh on Saturdays.

Over the next few months the ducks and swans would spend quite a bit of time in the garden amongst all the rubbish and rubble. They didn't even move away when we threw more stuff out – they would just waddle over to see if it was edible or not. Every few weeks we would borrow a trailer and get rid of all the rubbish from the house and garden and the ducks would be there waiting to grab the grubs and worms from under all the timber and the other stuff we moved.

As the weeks went on, the flat was beginning to take shape so we spent more time in the garden. During the summer months both Vic and I found it very hard to leave on a Sunday evening and go back to the school. The moon would be shining on the water and the swans and ducks would be preening themselves before settling down for the night. We would sit and talk about how we would like the garden and we drew up plans and looked at other people's gardens along the Widewater to get ideas. We agreed that we would wait until we had moved into the flat before we would start on the garden.

20th February, 1988, was a big day for me for it was not only the day we moved into our lovely home, but the day I celebrated my fortieth birthday. Life begins at forty, they say, and my head was bursting with ideas for the garden. The sun was shining that day and life looked really good from where I was standing. There was only one problem – because we had worked so many long hours on doing up our home while still working at the school during the week, I had become very tired. Not only that, a few months before we moved I had caught shingles from one of the children at school. I thought I was over it – if I kept working I would soon be back to my old self.

A month after moving I started work for one of our family friends and though I was always very tired by the end of the day, I believed that I would soon be well again. I only worked two or three days a week and the rest of my time was spent running the home or taking the boys to school or enjoying the garden. I would spend hours just sitting and watching the swans and ducks. They become very tame and I had changed their diet from bread to mixed corn, fresh water and as many slugs, snails and worms as I could find. Now the wildlife thought they owned half our garden so we had to redesign the whole layout and agreed that we would landscape the left side for our use and the right side would be for the ducks, so that was left grassed with just a few shrubs.

Our first summer came and went and we were all very happy in our new home. The boys had made plenty of new friends and Vic really enjoyed his job. My health was not getting any better but I was still happy. Autumn came and more ducks appeared on Widewater – they must have sent a message to all the wildfowl in the area that a new source of food had arrived since we had moved in. So instead of buying only a 7 lb bag of mixed corn each week, I was getting through a whole sack of corn over the same length of time. The cold damp weather was not making me feel any better and in fact my legs and arms were hurting and I found trying to work impossible. I was even falling asleep at work.

At Christmas we all went up to the Midlands to Vic's family for a short break. We had a really lovely time except that I was so tired – maybe I had overdone things in the last eighteen months. All the work on the flat might have been too much for me and I hadn't given my body time to recover from shingles properly. Well, I was still relatively young and I had always been very healthy in the past and I thought I just needed time – I would arrange to see my doctor when we get home. I was sure all I needed was a tonic.

4

Chapter Two

Once all the Christmas decorations were down and put away for another year, I felt eager to get back to work. I made an appointment with my doctor and tried to carry on as usual, but it wasn't that easy and the more I tried to do, the more tired I became. Even when I did nothing at all, I was still totally exhausted.

The day arrived to see my doctor and because I was a new patient he had to check my notes first. That didn't take him too long as the only times I had ever seen a doctor were when I was expecting the children and then I was a very healthy Mum-to-be. The last visit to my other GP was when he confirmed shingles fifteen months before. After I had told him all my symptoms he suggested a few blood tests and said I was at that 'age' when women get minor problems that are easily sorted out with hormones. This seemed like welcome news – I had too much to do to worry about my health. I had this wonderful new home, children that were becoming more independent and a whole new experience in wildlife waiting to be explored. I hadn't time to be ill.

I returned to my doctor time and time again because every single test was coming back negative. He went through all possible reasons why I should feel so very unwell and I was getting worse all the time. More and more symptoms were appearing, different from day to day, and I was becoming frightened that I might have a deadly disease.

When I started getting pins and needles down the right side of my body the doctor gave me a complete check over. It was when he started sticking a pin into my arms and legs that he realised it had nothing to do with my 'age'. With my eyes closed, all I could feel was the doctor's hand – I couldn't feel the needle at all. He left me lying on the examination couch and went to have a word with his partner. I didn't mind how long he was going to be as I was so tired I just wanted to go to sleep. They both agreed I needed to see a neurologist at Haywards Heath hospital, as the symptoms were very like multiple sclerosis.

For fourteen weeks I waited for the hospital appointment, by which time I had 'one foot in the grave'. Vic took the day off work to take me as I could no longer drive as the steering wheel was too heavy to turn. I saw a lovely lady doctor who made me feel very special and I was beginning to feel people were taking me seriously at last. The results of all these tests came back just like all the rest, negative. Was I really ill or was I going mad and imagining all these things?

No, I wasn't mad and after eighteen months of having tests and seeing specialists, I was diagnosed as suffering from myalgic encephalomyelitis (M.E.). It is a disease of the immune system. A virus had entered my body when I had shingles and from then on my immune system refused to work properly. I had an illness not many doctors believed in, let alone understood. Why couldn't I have had something else wrong with me that was curable?

The specialist advised me that I rest as much as possible. I was given painkillers and sleeping tablets, as there was nothing else they could do for me. The only positive help I was given was the address of Action for M.E., which is an organisation to help sufferers like myself. 1 wrote to them and they sent me a lot of information on M.E. – it was reassuring to know that I was not on my own with this disease and especially reassuring to know that I was not imagining it.

I soon had to give up work and I tried so hard just to rest, but it was out of character. I was told right at the beginning that there was no known cure at present and that I was to rearrange my life completely. I felt I had lost something so precious and that I wasn't going to get the chance of getting it back for a very long time. No one appreciates their health until they lose it. I couldn't just sit around all day – it wasn't normal – but I had no energy to do the garden and I had no energy to do any house-work. I couldn't even watch telly for very long before I became tired. I even tried doing jigsaw puzzles, but my brain wouldn't work. For nearly two years I sat around or tried to do something, but I only got worse. I didn't even have the strength to hold up the newspaper, I had to rest it on the table.

I soon needed a stick to help me balance and as I couldn't walk very far my doctor ordered a wheelchair for me. At first I wouldn't use it, I wasn't a cripple ... I wasn't old ... I wasn't mentally ill ... So why did I need a wheelchair? Then someone who does use a wheelchair, said 'Think of it as an aid to recovery, and that some days you feel well enough to go out in a wheelchair.' The first time we used it, Vic took me to Eastbourne for the day and I hoped I wouldn't see anyone I knew. But it was great. It was a hot summer's day and I had put on a dress with a v-neck front. My husband had a good view from where he was standing at the back of me. He said he would only push me if I wore something revealing. It was like using a carrot in front of a donkey.

We both enjoyed our day at Eastbourne and I wasn't as tired as usual, although pushing me made Vic's arms ache. It was only then that I realised that the whole family was suffering through my illness. It was years since we had all been out for the day together, because I wouldn't last the distance. But now I had the wheelchair, things were going to be different.

So now I had to learn to do things that would not drain all my energy, or make my arms and legs hurt. But what? Everything you do takes some degree of energy. All this time I had continued to feed the ducks and some days there seemed to be more than others. But I had noticed something strange – there were never any ducklings around. Come to think of it, there were only one or two female mallards on Widewater.

There is a lady who lives a few doors away, who moved to Widewater in 1933. She is a 'walking history book', but that's another story ... I asked her why there weren't any ducklings. She said there used to be at least eighteen pairs of swans and hundreds of ducks on Widewater all the time, but over the years the condition of Widewater had deteriorated and the wildlife had slowly dwindled. Also, there was a resident family of foxes on the north side of the lagoon and they never went hungry.

So, there were two major things that needed to be done. One was to restore the lagoon back to its former glory and the second was to encourage the wildlife back, but I had no idea of how to do either. It is funny how our lives take us on a path that proves to be the right one, but we don't think so at the time. Not only was I suffering from an illness that had no cure at the time; I was suffering from a sense of feeling totally useless and wanting to do so much but not having the energy to do anything at all.

Chapter Three

My life was to change for the better in spring 1990. It was
Winnie, our walking history book from a few doors away, who
phoned me early one day to say that our only female duck had
nested in her garden and laid seven eggs amongst the bluebells,
but sadly the fox had killed her and Winnie didn't know what to
do. She knew I was interested in the well-being of the wildlife so
thought I could help.

I went to see her right away as she had said the eggs were still
warm. Winnie had put them in a fruit basket and covered them
with some of the nesting material and a few of the mother's
feathers that were left lying around in the garden. All I knew
was that they must not get cold, so I took them home and put
the basket in the airing cupboard. Now what was I to do?

The only thing I could think of was to do what the children
did when they were in playschool when they sometimes had
chickens' eggs in an incubator ready for Easter. So I telephoned
all the schools in the town and was fortunate to find an
incubator that wasn't being used. I explained to the teacher
about my problem and she said I could use their machine. So I
went to collect it immediately as I didn't want the eggs to chill
too much. The staff were very helpful and loaded it into the car
as it was a heavy machine. They couldn't find any instructions,
but they did have the name of someone they knew who had
ducks, so they gave me his telephone number and wished me
luck.

I arrived home and a neighbour carried the machine indoors.
I plugged it in and switched it on then made the phone call

while the machine heated up. The gentleman at the other end of the line seemed very helpful and told me just what to do. So, with this new knowledge, I set to and once the incubator was at the right temperature, I went to the airing cupboard and gently picked up the basket of eggs and placed them onto the tray in the incubator. As I was putting them in I found myself talking to them – it seemed a natural thing to do. I talked to my own babies while they were in the womb so why not talk to eggs? An egg is a womb for birds.

I left a large note on my fridge door to remind me that I had to turn the eggs five times a day (one of the nasty symptoms of M.E. is memory loss). Another notice told me when to take my tablets and the other listed the times I had to turn the eggs. They made a good talking point whenever visitors saw them.

It takes twenty-eight days for ducks' eggs to hatch, so for twenty-eight days I would turn the eggs over, as instructed, and talk to them. Nothing much else happened as I didn't know what to expect. I had plenty of rest and I had collected some books from the library, to read up about ducks. On the twenty-eighth day I lifted the lid of the incubator and I saw that one of the eggs had started to crack. I gently picked it up and I heard the little duckling chirping. I nearly dropped the egg in surprise. I called Vic over to listen and then my son, Daniel. They agreed there was a noise coming from the egg. My sister phoned a little later to find out if there was any news on the eggs (I think I had bored everyone silly since becoming a broody hen). I was so excited that I put the egg to the phone so that she could hear the duckling. She said she could hear, but I think she was just being kind to her nutty sister.

Not knowing how long duck labour went on for, I was forever peeping in to see if anything had happened. But after two hours the egg was no further advanced. My excitement must have been catching, because my sister, Carol, turned up complete with video recorder for the event.

About six hours into labour another egg started to hatch and I went to get Winnie so that she could be there at the birth. The first egg that had cracked seemed too quiet and I realised that it must have died. The other five eggs seemed dead also, as they hadn't even started to crack. But number two was going well

10

and the more I talked to the egg, the more it tried to get out. So I kept putting the egg up to my face and giving the duckling words of encouragement. My sister and Winnie watched on but I had to keep the egg warm, so I put it back into the incubator. It was getting late in the day and Carol and Winnie had to go home, so I thanked them for the support and promised to phone the minute anything happened.

It wasn't until after they had gone home that I realised just how exhausted I was. Vic made me go and have a lie down, and seconds later I was asleep. I started dreaming about the egg, because I woke in such a panic when out popped a baby crocodile... 'No, no, you should be a lovely duckling...' Oh, thank goodness, it was only a dream.

It was now seven o'clock in the evening and there was very little movement from the only surviving egg. The only thing I could do and felt I should do, was to pick the shell off and help the poor little thing into the world. So, with a very steady hand I performed my first caesarean on an egg. With Vic and Daniel watching over me, I carefully picked the shell off until the duckling's head had emerged from the egg. Oh! he was gorgeous, a little wet head, big dark eyes and a beak that made the most wonderful sound. The tears were pouring down my cheeks. Both of my onlookers advised me to put him back into the incubator, as he could now breathe for himself, and have a rest again. I slept for about two hours and woke refreshed.

Surely he should be out of his egg by now, I thought, so I lifted the lid off the incubator and there in the corner lay the most wonderful sight – a very wet, exhausted duckling, minus his shell. I don't think my own labours were that difficult. My very patient and loving husband told me to let the duckling rest until the morning and advised me to go to bed for the night. It had been a very long day and I was shattered.

The next morning I went to see the little duck. What was wrong? He was just lying down with his legs sticking out behind him, as though he was flying. I knew he was alive because he tried to get up, so I lifted him out now that he was dry and he looked straight at me and started to chirp. I thought he must be alright if he was talking – but no, the poor little mite was deformed. What had I done wrong?

I knew of a charity called Wildlife Rescue, so I phoned them

11

up and a dear friend, Dave, came round straightaway as he lived only a few streets away. What he doesn't know about wildlife, he will always find out. He never gives up on any living creature.

He examined the duckling and agreed with us that his legs were deformed. This is caused when the egg does not hatch on time, so the little duck grows too big for his egg. Dave gave me the name of a lady who knows more about ducks than he does. She too, has become a very good friend to us. He said that there was a chance the duck could live, but he would need a lot of time spent on him, so I explained I had a lot of time going spare. I would have to feed him, using a fine paint brush with soaked chick crumbs on it and easing his beak open, get the food into him as, for some reason, he couldn't feed himself. He could drink when I held him and let him dip his beak into a glass of water.

His legs were a bigger problem. When Dave held the duck in one hand and eased his legs forward with the other, the duck could stand. But once Dave let go, the duck fell over. The only thing we could do was to massage his legs with baby oil and keep bringing his legs forward. This had to be done every twenty minutes, all through the day. Now, I could do that, so I got four little dishes: one for the food, one for the baby oil, another for his water and lastly one with eyewash in it. This was needed to clean the duck's eyes as he couldn't bring his feet forward to do it himself.

This was what I needed – to feel wanted and useful again, but not at this little fellow's expense. He needed all the luck in the world and a lot of courage. So we named him Plucky. For three whole days I did nothing else except care for Plucky. It was surprising how quickly twenty minutes kept coming round. I never had chance to have a sleep during the day, which I had been getting used to, but his needs were greater than mine. I kept Plucky in the incubator with the lid off. He needed the heat, and as he looked so uncomfortable I put him in one of my old woolly hats. I made it like a nest so that he could be propped up against the side so he could see all around him. Every time I came into his line of vision, he would begin to chirp away so happily. It was during the third day that Plucky was enjoying his water so much that he would dip his head deeper into the glass I was holding and splash the water all over his back. He was doing it so fast that all at once he went too deep and ... he was limp in my hand. Not a sound, not a movement.

I tried blowing into his beak, even rubbing his little chest to get life back into him. Nothing – he was gone and it was my fault, I should have been more careful. But he had been enjoying it and doing what ducks do, dabbling with water and now he was gone. Daniel was with me when this awful thing happened and he put his arms around me and we both cried.

When Vic arrived home he knew something was wrong and when we told him he agreed to bury Plucky in the garden. So we all went out there and laid him to rest. He had such a short life, but we shall never forget him. He helped to change my life and make me realise there is life with M.E. Thank you, Plucky.

Chapter Four

Losing Plucky like that did nothing for my confidence and for days after his death my health seemed to get worse. If only I could have turned the clock back to that fateful day, I would have paid more attention to what the duckling was doing. Both Vic and Daniel were wonderful – they told me there was nothing more I could have done for him. It might have been a blessing in disguise, because he may never have been able to walk, or keep his feathers in good condition, so that he would have become cold and unable to go in water and swim. Yes, it was a blessing – it would have been more cruel if he had lived.

The hatching of the eggs and the diagnosis of my illness happened at about the same time and my doctor became very interested in the ducks. I was visiting him every month as he was trying to get my medication right, and he was very sorry to hear about my loss. He realised how much it had upset me and told me not to give up and to try again. He agreed that it was a form of therapy for me.

Dave from Wildlife Rescue had given me the phone number of Sheila, who knew a great deal about rearing ducks, and about a week after Plucky died I rang her. It was a pity I didn't know her when I first used the incubator as things might have been different.

That afternoon Sheila came to see me, but she didn't come alone. In a box were four ducks' eggs. 'Dave told me what happened and we both think you ought to try again,' she said. Then she gave me a reassuring smile.

This lady deserved a cup of tea, so while I put the kettle on,

Sheila set up the incubator. But she set it at a different temperature, because I had it too low. Also, I turned the eggs the wrong way and I never sprayed them with water once a day. Well, as I hadn't been told that, it was no wonder six eggs failed to hatch. Over tea and biscuits we talked about ducks and nothing else. Sheila knew so much about them and she has was willing to teach me everything. Now, the reason you have to spray the eggs each day is to mimic the mother when she has been for a swim and then sat back onto her eggs. This stops the embryo from drying out. Sheila then showed me how to check the egg to see if it was fertile and alive. In a dark room you place a torch behind the egg and let the light shine through. If the egg is not fertile the egg will look clear; if there is an embryo inside you will see a dark patch. As the duckling grows inside the egg you can see it developing. Rather like a scan that mothers have, this process is called 'candling' and it is about the most exciting thing I have seen for a long time.

Sheila and I spent an interesting two hours together – we really got to know each other and we had so much in common. She promised to keep in close contact with me during incubation and would ring me regularly. I couldn't wait for it to get dark so that I could 'candle' the eggs. Seven days into the incubation period I knew that two of the four eggs were not fertile, so Sheila told me to take them out. The other two were doing well and, yes, I could see the little embryo growing. Once a day I would spray the eggs from a fine spray gun I used for my indoor plants. I used tepid water, so that I didn't frighten the growing embryo with cold water and I would also talk away to the eggs and tell them I was going to be their new Mummy.

About three days before the eggs were due to hatch I could hear one of the eggs chirping away. There was no sound from the other egg and Sheila said it must have died. I asked her why this happened and whether I had done anything wrong. She said that if all eggs that were laid subsequently hatched, then we would be overrun with birds. It was nature's way of keeping the numbers under control.

Not a great deal of housework was done while I waited for the big day. As I was getting a bit anxious, I found I was getting very tired, so if I wasn't talking to the egg, I was resting. I couldn't go to sleep during the day, but then no expectant mother sleeps very well at the end of her pregnancy. The more I talked to the egg, the more it got used to my voice, so when it did eventually hatch, the duckling would know who his mum was, by the voice. I am sure Vic was getting a bit worried about my behaviour towards the eggs and when he took me into a supermarket to do our shopping, he would keep me as far away from the shelves of eggs in case I started singing nursery rhymes to them.

The big day arrived. I couldn't wait and as soon as I got out of bed I had a peep in the incubator. Yes. yes, it had started! I went and woke Vic and Daniel. The fact it was only 5 a.m. was beside the point as most babies are born in the early hours.

I had been given a book called 'How to Incubate' by a family friend and on the front cover was a picture of three eggs hatching. The little bird pecks around the top of the egg until there is only a little bit of shell intact. Then it pushes the 'lid' off and pops its head out as though the shell had its own front door. Well, my little duck must have read the same book, because that is just what happened. At this stage the duckling was so exhausted that I let it have a long rest. If I hadn't been on medication I would have cracked open a bottle of champagne or, at least, white wine.

It took about another hour before the duckling was completely free from the egg and then it needed to dry out before I could take him out of the incubator. So I did some housework and popped across the road to get some shopping to keep myself busy. I knew I must not take him out too soon or he would get a chill.

Four hours after the duckling had hatched he was dry enough to be removed from the incubator. He was perfect, he could stand, his feet were facing the right way and he constantly quacked. He was a miracle and I had done it myself. I cannot describe the feeling, I couldn't take my eyes off him and he was beautiful. Well, all mums are biased, aren't they?

I sat in my chair, put the duckling in the woolly hat I had used for Plucky and gently laid my hand over the duck. The heat from that little bird was tremendous. Soon we were both sound asleep. I didn't wake up for nearly two hours and it was only when the duckling started to crawl from under my hand that I was disturbed. As I lifted my hand up two big eyes looked up at me and the duckling began to quack so loud, it was though he was saying 'Hi Mum, I'm hungry.'

I lifted the duck up to put him on the floor while I went to get some water and food. As I stood up, hundreds of tiny flaky bits fell from my lap. It looked just like my skirt was suffering from a bad attack of dandruff. It was the clear sheaths that cover each of the downy feathers – as the down dries, the sheaths drop off and resemble dandruff. I walked from the lounge into the kitchen to get the food and the duckling was right by my feet the whole time. If I moved forward, he was right there and wouldn't leave my side. As I stopped by the sink to get the water, the 'little ball of fluff' settled on my foot and started to peck between my toes, which really tickled.

I put a tiny dish on the floor with chick crumbs in it and another dish with water, but I made sure it wasn't deep as I didn't want him to drown in it. There was no need for me to show him what to do – he knew just how to eat and drink and make as much mess as possible, as quickly as possible. As he was doing so well on his own, I went to the other side of the kitchen to make a cup of tea, but he was right there, on my foot, pecking between my toes again. He had no intention of being very far from me. I was frightened of treading on him, so I put him in the pocket of my skirt and he settled down and went to sleep. I was able to walk around the house with him in my pocket and not worry about treading on him. As long as I talked to him and he quacked back, I felt he was happy. At least, I knew I was!

I found one of my old cardigans and when I sat in my chair, I put the cardigan down on my lap and put the duck in it, then draped one of the sleeves over him, like a wing, and he went to sleep quite contented. So I had my rest and felt very happy. I must have fallen asleep, because when I woke up, the little duck was not where I had left him. He had walked up my arm and had gone back to sleep on my shoulder with his head under my hair.

Later that day I had to get the family their meal, but every time I went to move away, the duckling quacked so much that, eventually, I had to put him in a box with my cardigan in it and leave him to protest. I talked to him the whole time so that he knew I hadn't deserted him and he seemed to accept that. He was a daft little thing, quacking all the time, so I named him Biscuit, because he was 'quackers' (cream crackers!).

While we sat at the table having our evening meal, Biscuit was going from one pair of feet to another until he decided that

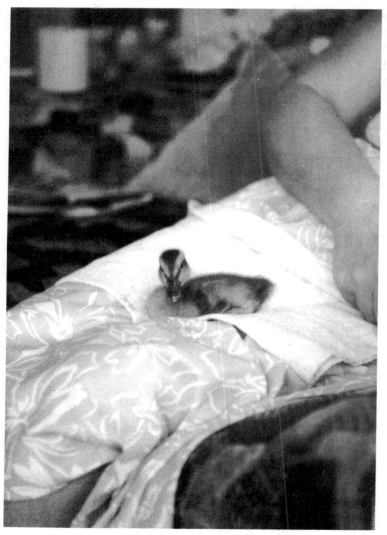

Biscuit and I having our afternoon rest together.

Vic had the warmest toes and went to sleep on them. Vic refused to take his socks off – he didn't want the hairs on his feet plucked out. During the evening I slept in my chair with Biscuit asleep against my neck, making noises in his throat the whole time just to let me know he was there. When we both woke up it was time for bed. It seemed to have been a very long day to me but I was so happy. Next problem was, how would Biscuit behave when left on his own? I put a hot water bottle under my cardigan in the box, then put the duck in and covered the sleeve over him again. 'Quack, quack, quack' was the result, but once the light was put out we never heard another sound out of him until daybreak at about 6 a.m.

Chapter Five

Next day, after I had washed and dressed myself and Biscuit had finished his breakfast, he started charging around the house with such confidence, it was hard to imagine that he was only twenty-four hours old. When it was time to wake Daniel up for school, I took Biscuit into his bedroom and put the duck on the bed. QUACK!!! QUACK!!! QUACK!!! – that soon woke him up!

I spent the day trying to do housework and cooking but it was so difficult when I had a duck trying to sit on my feet all the time. Twice he went sailing across the kitchen floor when I forgot he was on my foot, so he spent the rest of the day in my skirt pocket. After lunch I took him to visit Winnie. I carried him to her house, then knocked on the door. I put Biscuit on the ground and waited for Winnie to open the door. As she did so, Biscuit walked in unannounced.

'Well, who's your friend?' she asked.

We spent a lovely time with Winnie and Biscuit sat on her lap and snuggled under her warm safe hands and went to sleep. He was always either asleep or eating and already I could see a difference in his size. When he was on someone's lap he put his beak between their fingers, as though he thought they were that person's feathers. If the person squashed their fingers close together, he would force them apart with his beak. He also liked to be on my shoulder so that he could pull my hair or nibble my earring. It gave me goose bumps down my neck, or do I mean duck-bumps?

I had an appointment with my doctor a few days after the

duck was born. He said I looked much brighter and he thought the duck was a good tonic for me. My tablets were suiting me and I was coping with the illness. I was still seeing the doctor every four weeks but because I had such an interest in the duck, my illness wasn't getting me down.

When a female duck rears her own clutch, she sits on the young ducklings and her natural oils on her feathers rub off onto the young and make their down waterproof, so that very young ducklings can swim without drowning, within the first day or two. But hand-reared ducks like Biscuit have no oil, so I wasn't allowed to let him in deep water until he was four weeks old. By then he had lost all the down and had feathers and could oil them himself every time he preened.

The big day came for his first swim. The weather was lovely and warm, so I took the baby bath out into the garden and filled it with water, put a plank of wood on the grass and leant it against the bath. The whole time I was doing this, Biscuit was watching me and quacking his approval. Now, was I to pick him up and put him in, or let him walk up the plank and dip his toes in first? No need to worry – he went to the other end of the bath from the plank and climbed in with an almighty splash.

He took to water, as the saying goes, like a duck, and he splashed and dived. He cleaned every feather individually then ran down the plank, along the grass before charging back into the water. He did this for about half an hour until there was hardly any water left in the bath, and it was all in the grass. I was worried that he might get cold, but the water just rolled off his back in little droplets. He was completely waterproof and now that he had had his first swim, he was ready to swim the Channel. However, it seemed wiser to start with the Widewater!

Each day Biscuit grew bigger and stronger and he started to mix with the wild ducks. I didn't like the way he took longer to come to me when I called him. He was like a teenager and was starting to feel his independence. The days grew longer, so he spent more and more time in the garden and in the water. He was behaving like a proper duck and I was feeling a little jealous.

After Biscuit had hatched, I had returned the incubator to the school and thanked them very much for lending it to me.

Then, when Biscuit was about two months old, Vic came home from work with another incubator which he had bought for me as an early Christmas present (it was only July).

The duck was now nearly eight weeks old and was fully

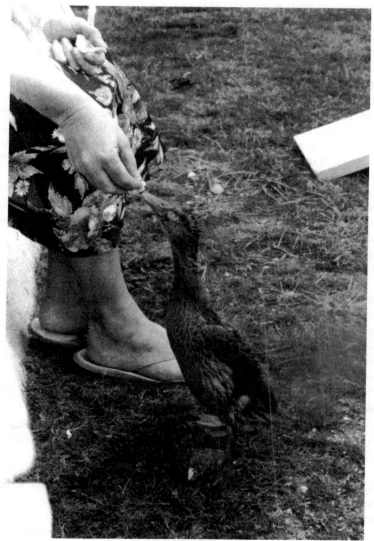

Biscuit and I sharing a lettuce leaf.

grown. They are not babies for long, so he started to sleep in the shed at nights. One very wet and windy night proved too much for the old door on the shed and it blew off its hinges. The wind was keeping me awake, so I got up to make a cup of tea and looked out of the window and saw the door hanging off. I got Vic to help me as I am not too good on my legs through my illness; the howling gale was making matters worse. We went down to the shed but we couldn't find Biscuit. I called to him but the wind was so noisy I wouldn't have heard him if he had answered. Vic secured the door for the night and I tried to see if our duck was in the water, but it was too dark to see. It was an awful night to be lost, especially as he had never been out all night before. Once Vic had made the door safe we started back up the garden steps and there by my feet was one very wet and soggy Biscuit. We took him indoors and dried him on an old towel, then left him to sleep on the kitchen floor.

Next morning I was greeted by a very lively duck and he was keen to get back out into the garden. I let him out and he went straight into the water with all the other wild ducks – that was when I realised that my job was over. I had done what all mother ducks do, watched my little duckling grow into an adult duck.

Whenever I went into the garden to put washing out on the line, or potter with my plants, or just sit in the garden, Biscuit would always come out of the water and sit by me. He would quack constantly, telling me what he and the other ducks had been up to. I hadn't yet seen him fly but he did try. He would flap his wings like mad and run along the water but he couldn't quite master it.

Biscuit loved his garden and he would help me do the weeding by picking out all the worms and getting rid of all the greenfly. He felt that he was safe in the garden, but that wasn't really the case: I wasn't able to teach him about the dangers that were around or about the foxes.

One morning, when my little duck was about three months old, I went outside to give him and all his friends their breakfast. A deathly silence hung in the air. A few ducks were in the water but none had come into the garden. I called to Biscuit, but I couldn't see or hear him. I went down to the water's edge to see if he was with some of the other ducks. But he didn't seem to be anywhere, so I was on the point of going back in to make breakfast, when I looked into my neighbour's garden and there he was.

On the lawn lay Biscuit, motionless, silent. The fox had been visiting gardens during the night, so he could feed his young. All the ducks, bar one, had sensed the danger, so had gone out into the water. Biscuit had gone into his garden for safety and that was his mistake. Going by the state of him he had put up quite a fight... That was my boy.

Later that morning I buried Biscuit in the garden. I felt sick about what had happened and annoyed with myself. I phoned my friend Sheila, and told her my sad news. She came to my house an hour later and we talked about the mistake I had made in keeping Biscuit too tame. I should have let him be with the wild ducks when he was old enough to swim – at four weeks old. Sheila stops handling her ducks and lets them learn from the older, wild ones.

I was in two minds whether to try again, but I had so much encouragement from Vic, Sheila and Winnie that I said that next spring I would have another go. If I had given up then, the knowledge that Biscuit had given me and the sheer pleasure I had had would all have been wasted.

Chapter Six

We keep our compost heap at the bottom of the garden, by the water's edge. It consists of garden rubbish and straw that we put out for the ducks to sit on. Contrary to belief, ducks do not like sitting on wet soil all the time – they will enjoy a muddy puddle or two, but when they want to rest, they like their bottoms to be dry. So around the garden I leave small heaps of straw for them and when it has become too messy, I put it onto the compost.

The two swans have been living on Widewater for about twenty-five years and most years they will raise a family. Quite often they would come into our garden to feed on bread and corn and some days they would stay on the lawn and sleep. We felt very honoured when they did this.

The same year that Biscuit was born, the swans chose to make their nest in our garden on the compost. We were thrilled and it was lovely to watch the pen as she rearranged the contents of the compost. The male, called a cob, would go along to people's gardens and pinch twigs to give to his mate, carefully placing them on the nest for her so that she could put them somewhere different. I think she moved every piece he gave her – she was in charge of making a nest, so, on principle, she moved his offerings.

Once the nest was to her liking, she settled down on it and had a rest. Her mate would keep guard in the water and he got very angry if the ducks swam too close. When the pen was satisfied that the nest was a good place for her eggs she would call the cob into the water and they would mate. I know it wasn't very polite to watch, but it was the most graceful courtship I have ever seen. He was so gentle with her and the dance that they did was just like synchronized swimming but on the surface.

Swans will mate one day, then the female will lay an egg the following day, then they will mate the next and so on, until she has anything up to eight eggs. When the female has decided she has laid enough she will start to sit and incubate the eggs. They take it in turns on the nest and when she wants to eat and freshen up the male gets on the nest and keeps the eggs warm for her. The minute she gets back on the nest she turns the eggs over – it is incredible that a bird as big as a swan can turn an egg so gently without cracking it. Then she goes to sleep and her mate goes back on duty, guarding her. It takes thirty-seven days to incubate swans' eggs, so it is just as well the male shares in the rearing of his family. Swans are different from male ducks who play no part in nest-making or incubating; they just do the chasing and mating and then they are off.

I would go down into the garden to feed the ducks and swans each morning and they didn't mind as long as I didn't get too close to the nest. The day the eggs started to hatch there was a lot of excitement: the cob made sure the ducks kept away and he swam up and down in front of the nest and seemed very anxious. I thought of giving him a large cigar to calm his nerves, but neither Vic nor I smoke.

As soon as the cygnets started to hatch, the pen stood up on the edge of the nest and picked up the empty shell and threw it out. It was while she was doing that, that I was able to have a look, making sure I wasn't too near. The cygnets were beautiful and fluffy and made the tiniest squeaky noise. Considering the fact that the female lays her eggs every other day and that it can be as much as fifteen days difference between the first egg laid and the last, all babies are hatched on the same day. Isn't nature clever?

The mother stayed on her brood until the next morning and when I went down to feed them, she was standing next to the nest so that I could see them all. They were delightful and were busy picking bits off the nest and trying to eat it. It had been built up quite high by the parents and I was wondering how the babies were going to get into the water. I would never have believed it if I hadn't seen it for myself: the mother stood up next to the nest and opened one wing fully; she then put the wing behind all of the babies and 'cupped' them into her wing before flicking them into the water in one go. Splash, splash, splash, went all eight of them, as they flopped into the lagoon.

Those cygnets fell into the water like tennis balls and just floated and bobbed about. After a few minutes the parents took their offspring for a tour of their estate. It was also to show them off, because they looked so proud of themselves. I felt very privileged to have been there and witnessed such a marvellous event.

Nature proved itself to be cruel again when, the following morning, there were two cygnets missing. A neighbour had seen the heron stalking the young, so we thought that he must have taken them. One day Vic and I saw the heron on the other side of the lagoon and he was eating a water rat, whole. So knowing what a heron can do, we had to accept the fact he had eaten the babies for breakfast.

The other six cygnets and their parents continued to swim up and down all day long and the babies were learning very fast. They did everything their parents did, so when Mum and Dad washed themselves, the babies had a go. It was lovely to watch them and when they tried to preen themselves when they were all in our garden, the cygnets kept falling over.

During the previous winter, Vic had started to dig a trench in the garden for a wall to be built and he was going to finish it in the summer. One day the swans and their babies had been in our garden and had spent quite a while cleaning themselves and then they had a sleep. I went to fetch Daniel from school and when we arrived home the swans had gone back into the water. I made a cup of tea while Daniel went down into the shed for something – he then came running in to tell me one of the cygnets had fallen into the trench. I went to get an old towel as I wasn't sure if he would be all grubby or bleeding, and we went back down to the trench.

I had never touched a cygnet before, so I didn't know if he would bite me or not, but when I saw him he looked so frightened. I gently laid the towel over his head so that he wouldn't panic and climbed into the trench to pick him up. He was ever so light in weight and so very soft and warm and

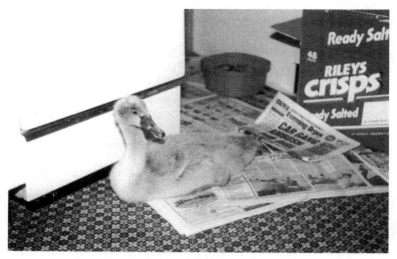

The cygnet rescued from the trench and waiting for Vic to come home.

although his legs looked rough, they weren't. I looked around to see if his parents were about, but there was no sign of them, so Daniel and I took him indoors.

I asked Daniel to put newspaper on the kitchen floor and then gently put the cygnet down and removed the towel. He stayed just where I had put him. I put a dish of water on the floor and then we left him alone for a while to get over his ordeal. I went and had my cup of tea and then discussed with Daniel what to do next. Vic was due home from work any minute and he always came in through the kitchen. I don't know who would have been more surprised, Vic or the cygnet, so Daniel wrote a note saying 'Beware, cygnet in kitchen' and went around and put the note on the back door to warn him.

We didn't have long to wait before we heard Vic's van come into the drive and he saw the note, so came in through the other door. We went into the kitchen to see if the cygnet was alright and he had got up off the floor and was wandering around and I could tell that he had drunk some water, which was good. Vic said the parents might not accept him back because humans had handled him, so what would we do if that happened? He said we must try and give him back before it got dark so I asked

30

if he would take a photograph of me holding the cygnet first, as this may be the only chance I'd ever have.

After the photo session I covered the youngster up in the towel and we all went out to find the swans. They were right up

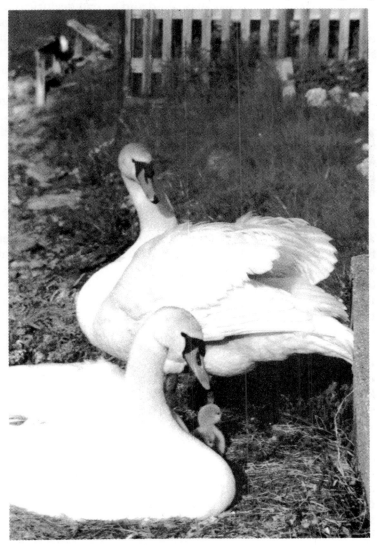

The proud parents

the other end which was too far for me to walk, so we drove in the van to the other side of Widewater where there was a car park. All the other swans were on the little island in the middle of the water, so we slowly walked to the water's edge. By this time the cygnet had grown all relaxed and he had his little neck hanging over my arm. The male swan soon saw us and he came over so fast I thought he was going to attack us. Vic told me to slowly put the cygnet on the ground and then stand very still.

The cob had his wings out in a fighting gesture and the cygnet realised it was his dad and swam out to him. As the baby got nearer, the cob put his wings down and turned to go back to the island and the little one followed him. His mummy was so pleased to see him and she made such a fuss, it was lovely to see. I was pleased that they had accepted the cygnet but I wasn't sure if they would ever come back into our garden – knowing one of their youngsters had fallen into a trench, they might not chance it again.

First thing the next morning I went out into the garden to feed the wildfowl and all the swans were there waiting for me. They had either forgiven me for putting their baby in danger, forgotten all about it, or their breakfast was more important. Whichever it was, I was pleased to see them and they continued to come to me to be fed all through the summer.

Chapter Seven

The weather was growing a lot colder and it had been three weeks since we had lost Biscuit. There were quite a few more mallards turning up each morning to be fed and I would look at them all, but none had Biscuit's colouring or mannerisms. He was, and will always remain, very special to me.

My health was not improving and the doctor was worried, so he made me an appointment to see a specialist at hospital. The muscles in my arms and legs were so painful that I found walking was becoming very difficult and I had no strength in my hands. I underwent many tests at the hospital but nothing was found. I was beginning to get depressed because I had now been ill for over four years and there was still no cure. I was also very frustrated that the media were calling my condition 'yuppy flu' and that name seemed to stick.

I have never been a yuppy or frightened of hard work, or even a hypochondriac. But all of us who suffered from this disease were having a very difficult time trying to prove that we were really ill. My dear doctor was so understanding and he did believe in me and M.E. One day I felt so very ill that I went to see him, only to find that it was his afternoon off. I had to see another doctor.

I sat in the waiting room for what seemed like hours, the seat getting more uncomfortable, and I just wanted to curl up on the floor and go to sleep. Then I was called in to see a locum doctor. He didn't believe in myalgic encephalomyelitis and made me feel a fraud. He said that after I had had shingles I had become weak, but now I was 'better' I had to wake my muscles up. He gave me a tonic and said I was to stop wasting the doctor's time with this make-believe illness and to get on with living and working, so I should start by going for a five-mile walk along the beach.

I don't know how I got home, my mind was in such a confused state. Was I only thinking I was ill? If so, why did I feel so tired after just getting up in the mornings? After making a pot of tea, I needed a rest before I had the strength to pour it out. Just walking across the road to the local shop left me totally exhausted and in pain.

So, I decided to prove I was really ill – I would go for that walk! They would see what would happen; they would find me collapsed on the beach and with a bit of luck the tide would be coming in and that would be that.

I was all ready to go out. I had my stick in one hand and the keys in the other and I had just reached the front door when the phone rang. Was I to answer it or not?

'Hello Linda, it's Sheila here, I am glad you're in; I have just been given a female mallard that is in such a bad state and she needs so much tender loving care, you are the ideal person.'

I thank God for that phone call – it stopped me feeling sorry for myself and from doing something stupid. But I never want to feel that way again – it was too easy to walk into the sea and that frightened me. Anyway, the people who know me, know I am really ill. There may not be a cure but that doesn't mean that the illness does not exist.

It was then that I knew why I had M.E. If I had been healthy, I would still have been going out to work and doing things I wanted to do. Now I was doing things for other people and wildlife. I had the ideal place for the sick or injured birds, but most important, I had so much time to give. What I was doing didn't use up my limited supply of energy and it suited both me and the birds.

Vic was so supportive. He fenced in the 'duck side' of the garden and dug a pond in it. We then bought some rabbit hutches and put them in the garden to be used as convalescent quarters, and I planted some shrubs that would give the birds natural surroundings. The mallard that needed TLC was soon well enough to be released and she is still living at Widewater three years later.

Chapter Eight

At last, spring arrived and all the daffodils and crocuses were enjoying the sunshine. The ducks were busy getting their feathers to look their best and the drakes were chatting up the few females on Widewater, who wanted to look their best. The two swans were doing their mating dance and I felt like putting *Swan Lake* on the record player to accompany them. They were so graceful and so devoted to each other. Swans mate for life; it is a pity humans aren't quite so dedicated.

I was feeling a lot stronger and I had started driving the car again. I couldn't drive far, about ten miles each way was enough, so I decided to go to a garden centre to buy a few more plants. Next to the centre was a smallholding and a notice there took my eye. 'Duck eggs for sale,' it said, '60p for 6.' Well, I couldn't resist. I drove into the entrance and there was a stall with some fresh duck eggs in boxes. The ducks were waddling around the farm as though they owned it. A very large, well-rounded farmer came over to me and I thought it best not to say what I was going to do with them.

'Mornin',' he said.

'Good morning. Could you tell me what sort of duck eggs these are, please?' I said. (I asked this because the ducks on the farm looked a bit of a mixture.)

'Well, them's duck eggs,' he replied.

I decided I couldn't insult him, so I purchased six duck eggs and handed over my 60p. If they weren't fertile, I wouldn't be wasting a lot of money. I then called in at the garden centre and bought some pansies and potting compost. On the way home I started talking to the egg box with the ducks' eggs in – I was eager to get the incubator back into business.

After a week I found, when 'candling' the eggs, that only one was infertile. Not bad for 60p! I was much more confident this time and was able to continue with my boring household chores and leave nature to get on with hers.

Bang on cue, on the twenty-eighth day the eggs started to hatch and in eight hours all five ducklings were successfully free from their shells. The first one to hatch was a lovely pale colour and had a very long neck so we called him Lofty. The second was very rounded (a bit like the farmer) and very dark except for a yellow chest (this will turn white when the feathers come). He had jet black legs and huge yellow blotchy feet. His walk was very strange, prompting Winnie's daughter-in-law to say that he walked like Max Wall. So he became known as Max. The next three to hatch looked like pure mallards.

Because these ducklings hatched together, they stayed very close to one another. I was only there to feed them, I still handled them a lot in the first two weeks, but once they started to feather up I kept them out in the duck run. They soon grew up to be fine-looking ducks, except Lofty turned out to be Loftetta and Max became Maxine. These two ducks were very friendly – their parents must have been domestic ducks. They would wonder indoors in the mornings and I would give them some lettuce leaves which was like giving children sweets. They would help me do the gardening and wait for me to hand them a worm or two. It wasn't long before Loftetta and Maxine found themselves being chased by some very passionate drakes. The first time I saw one of them mating Maxine I thought, 'How dare he, she's only a baby.' But ducks grow up very fast.

The following spring, Maxine made a nest in the garden and laid seventeen eggs. As I said, she was a big bird. She had been sitting on them for about two weeks, when the fox came. I'm sorry to say he killed her and took some of the eggs, leaving all the others broken. It is very hard to accept what goes on in the duck world, but it is nature – we are all here to be food for someone, some day.

I must admit I did enjoy the incubating. I found it very rewarding and it didn't take much of my energy. A lady I knew who reared free-range chickens and had a few ducks, asked me if I would incubate some chickens for her. All I had to do was hatch them out and return them to her when they were a week old. That was just what I needed. I drove over to her farm which was further away than I thought so it made me quite tired. As she was very keen to show me around, I spent a good hour with her. I had never realised there were so many types of chickens. I told her the size of my incubator and she said it would hold four dozen eggs.

'How many?' I asked, somewhat taken aback.

'Four dozen,' was the reply, and I would have to turn them by hand, five times a day. Oh well, in for a penny, in for a pound, as they say. I went to open the car boot while she collected the eggs. I moved the wheelchair to one side and she put two trays of eggs carefully down in the boot. I thanked her and said I would phone as soon as they hatched. 'Now don't worry if any of them break,' she said.

I have been driving for many years and I pride myself on being a careful driver. I was only a few minutes from home when a car shot out from a side road. I did an emergency stop, but my wheelchair in the boot, didn't. I pulled up at the side of the road and walked very slowly to the back of the car. I was dreading opening the boot – what was I going to find? Have you ever wished you could turn the clock back just thirty seconds? Well, at this moment, I did.

I lifted the boot lid and inside there were forty scrambled eggs swimming on the floor. I was only able to save eight eggs, so when I got home, even though I was totally exhausted, I had to clean the boot out. Daniel was at home by this time and when I told him what had happened, a very slight smile came over his face.

'What am I going to tell her?' I said to Daniel.

'Do what you have always told me, tell the truth?' he said.

I made myself a cup of tea and dialled her number. Her husband answered and said, 'What's up, broken them all have you?' How did he know? I then went on to explain. They were very good about it and I incubated the remaining eight eggs but only two hatched. Believe it or not, she gave me another twenty to incubate and I managed to get them all home safely. Eighteen of them hatched.

I took these eighteen chicks back to her farm and she asked if

I wanted any chickens for myself. I explained that I only kept ducks, so she offered me a couple of my choice. I had a good look round and in one duck pen there was a small duck sitting and facing the wall. She looked as if she had been naughty and the teacher had made her go and sit in the corner until she could behave herself.

'What's the matter with her?' I asked.

'Oh, she was born without any eyes,' was the reply. I asked what was going to happen to her and I was told that both she and her sister, who had bad feet, were being fattened up for the pot.

You have guessed it – I said I would like to have them. She couldn't understand why I had chosen those two when I could have had any other perfectly healthy ducks.

Once I was home I had a good look at my newcomers. They were apricot Call ducks, were very small in size and about four months old. The blind one had no eyes at all. The eye sockets were empty, but eighteen months later, they had healed over. We named her Little Nell and her sister is called Tootsie, because she has poorly feet – the skin was very dry and kept splitting, making her limp.

I put the two ducks in their garden and watched them. Little Nell just walked around in circles all the time until she bumped into something. Her sister was talking to her all the time – Tootsie found the food and water and called to her sister and kept on talking until she too found the food. It was wonderful to watch them; Tootsie was acting as Little Nell's eyes.

The blind duck didn't like going into the pond at first and she would spin round so fast that I thought she would make herself giddy. So I put some bricks in one end of the pond and put my hand at the back of the duck and led her to the bricks. Once she could feel the bricks, she climbed onto them and started to clean herself. She spent a long time on the bricks, then she used her beak like a walking stick and felt all around herself. When she was confident where she was, she climbed back into the water, had a swim around, then swam to the bricks and climbed out. My Grandad was blind and I feel that has helped me to understand Little Nell's problem.

It wasn't long before Nell could walk around her duck pen without bumping into anything. She doesn't even use her beak as a walking stick any more and it's so rewarding to see how happy she is. Even her sister's feet are getting better. It must be all the insects and worms in their diet that is helping them both.

When they were about six months old I noticed Little Nell had gone into a corner of her garden and was pulling up the straw around her – I normally leave this in heaps around the pen – as though she was making a nest. In fact that was precisely what she was doing. Once she was satisfied with it she just sat very still. I looked at her and she appeared to be concentrating – even though she had no eyes, there was a look about her that gave that appearance. It was quite a few minutes before she made a move and then she made a loud sound. What was wrong? My Little Nell had just laid her first egg. She stood up and examined it with her beak, turned it over and then sat back down on it. I swear she was smiling, she looked so pleased with herself.

Chapter Nine

It has been two years since I first became a foster-mum to so many ducks. Plucky is still very much in my thoughts and I thank him for giving me such a wonderful interest. It really has helped me with my illness, because I have to get up every morning and feed all the ducks, no matter how ill I feel. Once I am in the garden and all the ducks come running round me, asking to be fed first, all my own needs are forgotten. The doctor always asks after the ducks as he knows how much they help me.

One morning I opened our local weekly paper and saw an advert in the pet section: 'Male duck needs good home, our garden not large enough, £3.' So I telephoned to find out more. He was a large duck and the only water he had was in a washing-up bowl and he couldn't swim in it. The owners also had chickens and this duck was getting frustrated and drowning the chickens in the bowl. I said I could give him a good home, so they agreed to bring the duck to me at the weekend.

During the week we had so much rain, the garden became very much like a mud bath, which the ducks loved. The couple came over with their duck, the husband carrying such an enormous box that I wondered just how many ducks he had got in there. He placed the box down carefully on the grass and opened the lid. I had never seen such a large duck. He was beautiful. He had the same colouring as a male mallard but he was at least four times bigger. They said he was a large Welsh Harlequin and his name was Whistler. He was so friendly, I fell in love with him, and as I lifted him out of the box, I was surprised how light he was – I thought he would have weighed a ton.

He had a good look around and when he saw the Widewater, he ran down the steps and jumped straight in. Splash! Admittedly, he was a big duck but he should not have sunk, which is what started to happen. I went into the water and got him out. He didn't seem to have any oil on his feathers and he resembled a very large drowned rat.

We had had so much rain during the week, the duck had got filthy, so the lady had decided to give Whistler a bath in washing-up liquid before bringing him to me. I had to put the duck in the shed so that he wouldn't get cold. When the couple left, I phoned Dave at Wildlife Rescue and asked his advice.

I had done right by getting him out of the water quickly, and I was to leave him in the shed until he had preened himself and got oil back in his feathers. It took four days, but then he was keen to get back into the water. He loved it and it was good to see the water rolling off his back in droplets. I don't think he came out of the water for about three hours – he was so happy, he cleaned himself and dived and splashed. It was a wonderful sight.

Whistler was a very happy duck and he never attempted to fly away or leave Widewater. Every morning he was by our front door waiting for his breakfast. Between our flat and the garden is a footpath, approximately four feet wide and thirty-three feet long. Whistler decided he owned it and if any other duck came near, he would see it off – even the seagulls got their marching orders! If we had any visitors he would stand and watch and give the impression that if anyone stepped out of line, they would come off worse, but with the family he was gentle and we all loved him.

If he wasn't having a swim he would be on patrol along his footpath or asleep on it, with one beady eye open. He was very possessive about his path but it seemed right that he should own something as grand as a path as he gave the appearance of having some royal blood in his veins.

A few months before Whistler arrived, I had hatched out four eggs that Loftetta had left lying around. One of the ducklings was a lovely blonde colour and tall like her mother. When she

42

was four weeks old, Sheila asked me if she could give it to her brother as a gift. I had no objection to her having any of our ducks as she had been so helpful and I didn't want to be overrun with them.

After Blondie had been with Sheila's brother about two months, it was clear that she wasn't happy. He already had two males and they wouldn't leave her alone, so he asked if I would take her back. I put her in the duck run with Little Nell and Tootsie until she had settled down after the move. She seemed very happy to be back and was soon picking out grubs, worms and greenfly. One lovely warm afternoon I was sitting on the step at the top of the garden. It has become my favourite place, because I have a good view from there and I can sit for hours watching the ducks, which ensures that I have a lot of rest. Two or three hours can disappear in a twinkling when watching the wildlife.

Blondie was at the top of the duck run, eating away, when Whistler came back from a swim. He usually has a drink of fresh water, which is always available, and then waddles up the steps to the top of the garden and then back on patrol along his footpath. However, today, he was drinking his fresh water, then looked up and saw Blondie, looked down again to drink then shot round for another look. It was love at first sight. He made such a noise and ran up the steps, two at a time, for a better look. Blondie looked up at him and she too made a strange noise. Whistler pressed his beak up against the netting that was separating him from this most wonderful duck. I had to get Blondie out of the duck run before Whistler did himself some damage.

I gently put Blondie down on the step that I had been sitting on and Whistler stood as tall as he could, sticking his chest out as far as he could to make himself look like a Chippendale. I swear he sighed – he was in love. He walked up to her and started to clean her feathers for her and she, like a lady, sat down and let him continue this ritual. After a while, Whistler took Blondie for a walk along HIS footpath. He even picked worms for her. If only I had a video, I could have recorded this unbelievable sight. I never knew ducks could be so passionate.

Every morning I would go outside and there would be Whistler and Blondie; they never left each other's side. I would put food down for them and Whistler would let his mate eat first like a real gentleman. Once, I threw them a lettuce leaf and they both picked it up, one each end, and then munched away until they met in the middle. I was expecting him to give her a kiss, as they had begun to resemble humans so closely.

Over the next few weeks their relationship grew stronger and they started to mate. Even in that, Whistler was gentle, unlike the wild ducks in the water who were on, off and away. There was nothing like that with Whistler. Then one day, two light-coloured males turned up. They walked up onto Whistler's footpath and while one pushed Whistler away, the other mated with Blondie. Then they swapped over and did it again. Whistler went mad. He bit the two newcomers and soon made them go, but for the next few days they came back and repeated their actions.

One day, I got so cross with these two strangers that I went out and picked them both up and threw them back into the water. Whistler seemed to appreciate that. Blondie soon decided it was time to make her nest and chose a quiet corner of the garden, right by my wishing well ornament. Vic had fitted a green bulb into the roof of the well many years before and in the evening when it was switched on, it looked very romantic. So it was the right place for Blondie and she would sit on her nest and Whistler would be on the lawn as near to her as possible. It wasn't long before she started to lay her eggs. Whistler continued to mate with her, but so did the two 'Bovver Boys', as I called them.

Blondie laid thirteen eggs over a period of days and then started to incubate them. The Bovver Boys never came back and I never ever saw them on the Widewater after that. Whistler stayed with Blondie, guarding her and her eggs. I put food and water out for her and he never left her side. I prayed that the fox would not come, and each morning I would sigh with relief when I saw them both safe and sound in the garden.

It was about a week before the eggs were due to hatch that I noticed Whistler was not on duty. I looked around for him, but he was nowhere to be seen. Blondie was sitting tight on her nest, so I left some food for her and then went to feed the others on the water. There, at the bottom of the garden was Whistler. He was dead. I asked Dave to come and see him and he said the duck had died of old age. I never knew how old he was when I got him, but I know he died a happy duck.

Blondie was too busy with her brood to notice he was missing, at least I hoped that she was. On the big day she hatched eleven of the eggs – even ducks can't get thirteen out of thirteen. The ducklings were lovely, but every one was light in colour, just like Mum and the Bovver Boys. Whistler had been firing blank bullets, but never mind – he was happy thinking he was the father.

A student who lived a bit further along Widewater had shown a lot of interest in my ducks and asked if he could have a go at rearing some of his own. So when Blondie moved from her nest, the day the eggs hatched, I took two out of the nest and gave them to Paul. He was so pleased and he successfully raised these ducks into adulthood.

On the second day Blondie took the babies for a swim and it was wonderful to see nature doing her job. Each evening she would make them get back on the nest for the night. I just wonder whether she thought Whistler had deserted her – I hope not. Each day the ducklings grew stronger and Blondie proved to be a very good mum, spending hours teaching them to hunt for insects and worms. The grass was never very long, but to watch a duckling chasing a fly and having to struggle through blades of grass that were as tall, if not taller, than himself, was a comical sight.

As the ducklings became more adventurous, they would spend longer in the water. The mum would be swimming gracefully along with all nine following in a straight line behind her. One day, after a very busy swimming lesson, Blondie came back into the garden and up the steps to do some more fly-catching. The children followed behind her, but there were only eight. As ducks can't count, she was not at all worried, but I could hear the duckling making such a fuss. I went looking for it. It wasn't far away – because they had been swimming a long time, this little fellow was too tired to climb the steps. He was so exhausted that he couldn't jump high enough to get up them. So I picked him up and carried him to his brothers and sisters. I could see why so many ducklings didn't live long in the wild: if one strays away, the mother will not wait or go back for it. You keep up or you don't survive.

When the babies were six days old, I went out to feed them and I couldn't see them anywhere. They were not by the nest where they usually were first thing in the morning and since I couldn't see them in the water either, I assumed they were getting braver and more adventurous. I fed the other ducks and treated Little Nell and Tootsie to their morning lettuce leaf, when the telephone rang. It was Winnie. She seemed very upset. She didn't want to worry me but she could see a pile of feathers in her neighbour's garden and they were the same colour as Blondie.

I went straight round there and my heart sank when I saw what had been a very special mother duck. She must have put up such a fight and there were feathers everywhere. But where were her babies? I knew it had been the fox, as foxes don't seem to care whether they are killing someone's mum; a duck is a duck to a fox.

Winnie and I looked everywhere for the babies, desperately hoping the fox hadn't killed them as well. As it was a windy day, the noise of the sea and wind made it difficult for us to listen out for the ducklings. I am an animal lover, but at times like this, my loyalties are on the side of the duck.

We kept on looking, but there was no sign of them. I telephoned Paul, who had the two ducklings, but he hadn't seen the other babies. I couldn't just leave it, so I went back home, put on my Wellington boots and went into the water. It is very soft mud at the bottom of Widewater, so I had to be very careful. The water might only be three feet deep in places, but the mud must be deeper, and I can't swim.

At first I thought it was just wishful thinking, but I was sure I could hear something. I moved carefully along in the water and the noise got stronger. Yes, I was right – it was the babies. They had hidden themselves under the upturned boat at the bottom of a neighbour's garden. As soon as I went near them, they started to panic. Why should they react like that to me? It was only the day before that I had been sitting on the top step with two of them asleep on my lap.

Whatever had happened during the night had upset them terribly and although I will never know for sure, I can guess. I realised I was not going to be able to catch the ducklings on my own, so I telephoned for Dave. He came over with his canoe

46

and catch-net. He was able to paddle out into the water and corner the ducklings by a little inlet on the other side of the lagoon. He carefully put the net over them and lifted them into the canoe, but there were only six ducklings. Three were missing.

Dave gave me the six and then went looking for the others. He never found them. He spent nearly an hour looking, but they too must have been killed by the fox. On that fateful night, I think Blondie knew the fox was around and swam away from the ducklings so that the fox would follow her, but three of the little ones must have gone after her. All I know is that the remaining ducklings were very frightened and whenever I went near them, they would try and hide.

I took them into the house and made up a warm bed for them in a large box and then covered it with a blanket. They must have been exhausted for they were soon asleep. It took about a week to gain their confidence but they were never the same little innocent ducklings again. They always stayed very close to one another, so when they were three weeks old, I put them in the duck garden with Little Nell and Tootsie.

They took one look at Little Nell and thought she was their mum. The fact that she was less than half Blondie's size didn't seem to matter as they went by the feather colouring. Poor Nell wasn't too happy with this fan club of hers and kept trying to run away. Gradually she started to talk to them and they all agreed that Nell would be like an auntie, and no more. Soon it all calmed down in the duck garden and it wasn't long before the ducklings were much bigger than Nell and her sister. They didn't need an auntie any more and I am sure Nell was relieved – she enjoyed laying eggs but not caring for the contents.

When the six orphans were fully feathered, I let them out of the run and they soon settled on Widewater. They were bigger than mallards but they all had Blondie's colouring. Paul telephoned to say he too was going to release his ducks onto Widewater and would I look out for them. Considering his two ducks were given to him on the day they hatched, I was surprised to see them in my garden within an hour of being set free. It was as though they knew that their brothers and sisters lived here. They all met up and are still together to this day – you would think that Paul's two had just popped out for a

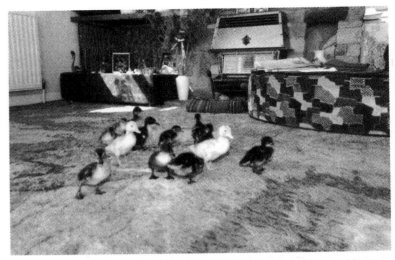

Some of my ducklings in the lounge. They are four days old and already fun to watch.

minute and then come home. It must be a very strong bond that wildlife have.

I know I am an old sentimentalist, but I like to think that Whistler and Blondie are together in heaven looking down on their family and feeling very proud of themselves. I bet that if there is a footpath by the Pearly Gates, it is being patrolled by Whistler, Blondie and their three little offspring.

I hope you don't think that all my ducks have been killed by the fox. When I started rearing ducks, there were just eight mallards on Widewater. Now, three years later, there are about seventy, give or take a few. They are not all mine – some have flown in and liked the area and have decided to stay – but there are at least forty ducks still living on Widewater that I have hatched and reared myself. It is the nesting mothers that are sitting targets for the fox. We are going to have to do something to protect them next year, because, now the numbers are up, I would like nature to do her share of incubating, leaving me to concentrate on caring for the sick and injured ducks.

Chapter Ten

Our family of swans was doing very well. The six cygnets were the same size as their parents now and the only way you could tell them apart was through the colouring – the young ones still had some brown feathers and their beaks were still black (they turn orange when they become adult). They were about five months old and they spent many hours learning to fly. It was a very funny sight when they ran along with their feet slapping the water and their wings going nineteen to the dozen, but they just could not take off.

The male swan was giving the children another flying lesson, when, overhead he heard the flapping of swans' wings. He looked up and there were two adults just above them who were getting ready to land. Straightaway the cob fanned out his feathers to make himself look twice his size and then travelled at such a speed towards the intruders that he was causing quite a wash. The mother swan stayed with the babies while the father went to battle.

When a swan is trying to chase away another one, he has to make himself look menacing, but to humans, he looks even more regal and elegant. His feathers are fanned out so that he can move through the water at a great speed, then he lays his neck back between his wings. Winnie has described this action as being like 'a galleon at full sail'. It is a magnificent sight.

The two intruders thought they were entitled to be on Widewater so they decided to fight for it. Our mother swan and her babies just stayed still in the water and watched. The other

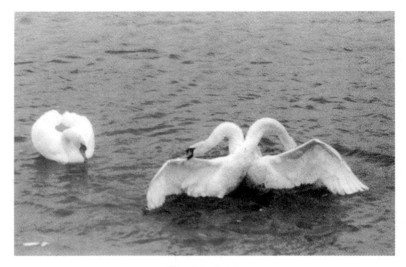

The big fight.

female didn't interfere but watched from the edge of the water while the two males fought it out.

At first I thought this was going to be a fight with half a dozen three-minute rounds and then the intruders would go, but not this time. It was horrible and both Vic and I realised that they

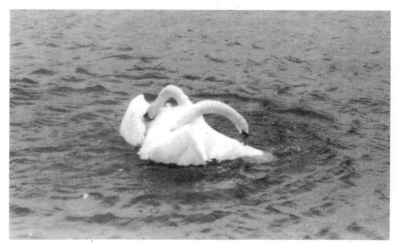

Our male swan is losing the fight with the intruder.

were going to fight to the bitter end. The noise they were making brought our neighbours out to see what the fuss was about. They started shouting at the swans to stop and throwing small stones near them to put them off, but they carried on fighting as though nobody else was around.

Over the years we have seen the swans in one or two brawls but nothing like this. They wrapped their necks around each other and while still holding this grip, each one tried to break the other one's wing by biting the 'elbow' part of it. When that didn't work, one would get on top of the other and hold the opponent's head under water to drown it. The noise of their wings thumping the water was frightening and I was beginning to cry from sheer frustration of not being able to stop them. Vic went and fetched the hose thinking that if he squirted them with water it would give the loser a chance to get away.

The bottom of the lagoon is thick mud and the fight was causing the mud to be churned up and the swans were getting so black that we didn't know which one was ours. All this time the female swans and babies just looked on and I could imagine the children shouting, 'Go on Dad, kill him'.

One of the swans was able to get away and started to head for the land on the other side of the lagoon; it was chased by the other one, who wasn't going to let him go. When they both

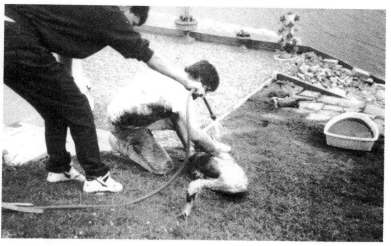

Dave and Daniel clean the swan before treating the wounds to his wing.

51

climbed out, it was obvious that they were exhausted and, because swans cannot move fast on land, they looked fit to drop. The swan that reached the land first was then knocked to the ground by the other one who then climbed on his back. Then he lifted the swan's head off the ground with his beak and thumped it hard down again. This went on four or five times and you could see the one on top was winning the battle.

Vic had run round to the other side of the Widewater and taken a broom with him in order to separate them without getting hurt himself. Before Vic got there, a man who was out walking, saw what we were trying to do, so ran down the bank, and with his hands waving in the air, he shouted as loud as he could. This worked and the two swans separated and the loser slowly walked to the water and the other one went the opposite way. I think they were both so tired that the fight would have finished soon anyway.

The intruder and his mate swam away to the far end of the lagoon and our female and her children swam away and left her mate to try and clean himself up. While all this had gone on, Vic had taken photographs of the fight – no one would have believed us if they didn't see the pictures. I never want to witness a fight like that again.

Our neighbours went indoors because the fight had really upset them, so we decided the best thing was to leave the swans to recover and contact Dave at Wildlife Rescue to let him know there had been this battle and to warn him that one of them might be injured.

It was about half an hour later that I looked out into the garden and I would have sworn that we had a black swan on the lawn. He wasn't just dirty but black, all over. The mud was dropping off the swan's back like thick black oil and that is what I thought it was at first. I went out to him and he went to flap his wings and blood splashed everywhere – it went all up the wall, over the grass and over me. He had been badly injured and it was then that I realised he was our swan. He had lost a fight for the first time and he looked so weak. I was able to get right up to him and he didn't make any attempt to object.

Dave soon come over to us and he had with him what looked like a strait-jacket for swans. He asked us to get the hose ready, which Daniel did, then Dave walked up to the swan, who just stood there, and put his hands around the bird's neck. The poor bird had no energy and Dave lowered its head to the ground and asked me to hold it for him. While I did that, Daniel turned the hose on and Dave sat astride the swan and very carefully lifted the injured wing. There was a nasty gash which was bleeding badly, so Dave said he would clean as much of the mud off as he could, then take the swan home and stitch up the injury.

As Daniel held the hose over the swan I held the bird's head with one hand and then with the other I stroked his neck and spoke calmly to him. Dave gently washed the mud off as he needed to see if there were any more injuries and it was easy to do it while we were helping. It appeared that the only wound was to the wing, so Dave slipped the strait-jacket over the swan and tied it firmly so he couldn't struggle and do more damage.

The swan was then put into Dave's car and he took him home. Vic, Daniel and I then cleaned up the garden where there was blood and mud over the grass and wall. We hosed it all down and waited for news from Dave. About two hours later the swan was returned to us with fourteen stitches under his wing – the other swan had made a hole in his side just where the wing joins the body. Dave asked me to keep an eye on him, explaining that he had given the swan an injection and that he should be put back on Widewater because he needed to be near his family.

Our poor swan stayed in the garden for ages cleaning himself and he perked up only with the return of his family. They all spent the rest of the day in the garden and there was no sign of the other swans so I hoped they wouldn't be back.

It was a week later before the male swan was fit enough to go out into the water and continue to teach his children to fly, but he never seemed very strong after the fight. He would spend hours on his own. I imagine it hurt his pride to think he had lost a fight in front of his family, but to me he was still champ. Dave told me that the swan came to our garden when he was injured because he knew he would get help and that made me feel good – I knew then that the wildlife trusted me.

Chapter Eleven

Little Nell and her sister, Tootsie, have settled very well in their garden, a large area measuring 12ft × 30ft which is fully fenced in, so any bird in there is safe from the fox. There are now three large rabbit hutches and a fair-sized pond in the duck garden which has clean water in it every day. If I am given a sick or injured duck or seagull, then it goes in the duck garden until it has recovered.

Vic and I decided that the duck garden needed a name of its own. We used to get confused when talking about the 'garden' – was it ours or the ducks' we were talking about? So it is now known as the 'Quackery'.

Any bird living in the Quackery has a good view of Widewater and all the wildlife on it and is never far away from its natural surroundings. Birds that are 'stressed' will not make a good recovery, so to help them I had to ensure that their convalescent home was right. I had also planted quite a few shrubs, so there was plenty of shelter in the hot weather.

I have had Little Nell and Tootsie for nearly two years now and Nell knows every inch of her garden. I always leave the drinking water and food bowls in the same place. She gets around at such a speed, hardly ever bumping into anything, that I sometimes wonder if she really is blind. The first year I had these two ducks, they laid over one hundred and fifty eggs between them, and as they had never mated, we used the eggs in cooking. The ducks were fed on mixed corn and their eggs tasted like chickens' eggs, which made them super for omelettes and sponge cakes.

Tootsie's feet have got better and she is a lovely looking duck. However, at one time I thought we might lose her. After she had moulted, I noticed her skin was very dry. Moreover, she had stopped going in the pond to wash herself, and the feathers that did grow were in a bad condition. I asked Dave to look at her, but he didn't know what was wrong, so suggested I made an appointment to take her to the vet's.

I bought a pet-carrier, normally used for carrying cats or any small animals, which was ideal for a single duck. So, when it was time to take Tootsie to the vet I went into the Quackery to get her. She must have known what was coming, because she was hiding and it took me ages to find her and when I did, she was behind one of the shrubs lying very low under the leaves. Once she was in the carrier we set off for the vet.

In the waiting room were a variety of humans and their pets. On one of the chairs a little old lady sat very quietly. On her lap was a small dog who looked very worried. I sat down opposite her and smiled and she nodded her head in acknowledgement but didn't look as though she wanted to talk. Next to her was a small child who was carrying a carrier just like mine. I didn't think she could have had a duck in hers somehow – she looked too normal (I have got used to people saying I am mad where my ducks are concerned). It proved to be a young kitten and when the girl smiled at me, I asked her its name. It was called Kitty and he was due for his injections. I told her they wouldn't hurt him, but she didn't seem convinced.

Next to me was a gentleman with a shoe box on his lap. Somehow I didn't think that his shoes would have been ill, so I assumed he must have had a small animal in it. There was no sound coming from the box, so I started to try and guess what he might have had in it. When the receptionist called over to him and asked how old the rat was, we all looked a little uncomfortable and were glad when he was the next to be called in to see the vet.

Tootsie was sitting very quietly in her box and I was wondering what she was thinking about, when in walked a man and lady who were both rather on the large side and seemed to take up the whole of the doorframe as they entered. Behind them they were dragging in an equally large dog who had no desire to see the vet that day or any other day. He was pulling on his lead and then barked in protest. Everyone in the waiting room held tightly to their pets. I was surprised that Tootsie hadn't made a fuss – she just sat very still in her box. Then the large dog, who started dribbling, began to cry. He didn't want to be at the vet's, so he cried and cried, then when his master shouted at him, he started to shake from head to tail. What a wimp!

It wasn't long before the old lady and her dog were called into the vet, followed by the little girl and her kitten. Soon it would be our turn. I just hoped the dog wouldn't find out what I had in my box. Could you imagine the chaos that would have caused? At last my name was called and in I went.

The vet was a very nice man and said he didn't have many 'duck' patients. With his clientele I didn't think this surprising! He gave Tootsie a thorough check over and said he wasn't sure what was wrong with her. He told me to try an antibiotic and see how she progressed; I was to wait in the waiting room for the medicine. A few minutes later he came out with a small container of yellow powder. I was to give Tootsie 5 mg. twice a day, and in order to do this he gave me a syringe with a small piece of plastic tube. I was to mix the powder with water and put it in the syringe, then get Tootsie's beak open and pull her tongue out as far as possible so that the tube went past her windpipe. In this way, I was to administer the medicine – if it went down her windpipe she would drown. This sounded like a hazardous undertaking.

There was no way was I going to do it on my own, so I phoned Sheila to ask her advice. She came over and showed me what to do. She made it seem easy, but it wasn't. When Vic came home, Tootsie was due for her second dose so we got her on the kitchen table on newspaper and Vic held her firmly. I opened her beak and tried to grab her tongue, which was slippery. Once I had a firm grip, I then had to pull the tongue out until the windpipe was in view. I was not enjoying myself, but managed to get the syringe past the pipe. But, as the medicine was going down, she pulled her head away in protest and spat it out all over Vic.

Well, after about four more attempts, we mastered it. It did get easier after a while, but then Tootsie decided she didn't want any more and would not let me open her beak, let alone grab her tongue. She would just sit on the newspaper and no matter how I tried, she refused to open her mouth. The vet said if her skin was improving then I should stop the treatment. Luckily her skin was better, so she didn't need any more. Now, whenever I go into the Quackery, she gives me an old-fashioned look and walks away holding her head down and her beak tightly shut.

Her skin really did improve and once her new feathers started to come through they were feathers to be proud of. Now she goes into the pond and washes herself daily – well, a girl has got to look her best. My father needed some antibiotic soon afterwards and I offered to give it to him through a syringe, but he wouldn't let me. I wonder why!!

Chapter Twelve

At the beginning of summer 1994 I had a telephone call from a lady called Sylvia who also helps to run an animal rescue. She had been given a duckling the night before and she had heard that I reared them without too much trouble, so I went to see her later that morning. She lived in the same town as me and I was glad about this because I wasn't feeling too good and I didn't fancy doing too much driving.

When I arrived at her house she invited me in and I could hear someone calling her, but she took no notice and started to make a cup of tea. This person, who was calling, was getting a bit annoyed at being ignored, but still she continued making the tea. Sylvia invited me to have a sit down and passed me a cup. 'If you like, I will show you round before you go,' she said, still ignoring the irate person in the other room.

I had my tea and was eager to get going as I didn't want to get involved in a family argument. 'We will start in the lounge and then go into the garden,' Sylvia informed me. Good, that should sort the other person out, I thought.

As we went into the lounge, there, in a very large cage was a very noisy mynah bird, shouting his head off and demanding his breakfast. Sylvia told me to ignore him as he went on like this when someone came to visit. I was so relieved and I need not have rushed my cup of tea after all. There were birds of all types in different sized cages and they were all in her lounge. There were birds with broken wings or legs and there was even one bird with a broken beak, but they all looked happy and well cared for. The mynah bird had a growth on his side and it was being drained – pity they couldn't do something about his voice box and manners!

In an incubator on the far side of her lounge was the tiny little black duck that I had come for. It certainly was not a mallard for it was very dark and had a short beak. I picked it up and held it firmly in my hands; it was shaking like a leaf. 'He was brought in late last night and he has not eaten anything yet,' explained Sylvia. Apparently a lady was taking her dog out for its evening walk, when she heard a crow scream as it flew overhead. She looked up and as she did so, the crow dropped what it was carrying. The dog ran after the object and the lady followed. Carefully the dog picked up this black 'thing' and gave it to his mistress – it was the duck that I was now holding in my hand.

It was amazing that the poor little thing hadn't died of shock but he was quite settled in my hand and was soon asleep. We then went outside to see all the birds that were too large to be indoors. There were at least ten seagulls and lots of pigeons. I stayed for only a short while because I wanted to feed the little duck. After all it had been through, it would have been a shame to lose it simply because it hadn't anything to eat.

As soon as I arrived home I put the duck in a box with a hot water bottle and my old cardigan. That cardigan has certainly come in useful! I fed the duck and then let it rest while I looked through Vic's book *Ducks of Britain*. I discovered that our little newcomer was a tufted duck. It was smaller than a mallard and would dive for its food; when fully grown it would be black, with a white belly and a tuft on its head. I named it Tufty as I couldn't think of anything else.

Tufty grew very slowly and it made a nice change to have a different sort of duck to look after. He loved to dive in the pond and could hold his breath for a long time. When Tufty was eight weeks old we discovered that 'he' was a 'she', so we kept the name but we now realised that we needed a mate for her. I contacted a duck breeder and asked if they had any male tufted ducks for sale. They had, so Vic and I went and bought a mate for our Tufty. He cost us £22.50 which I thought was rather expensive, so I was glad that our duck liked him or there might have been trouble (for me, that is). The male duck had very bright eyes, so that became his name. Bright Eyes and Tufty have been very happy together and I hope next spring they will mate. I can then sell the babies when they are older and get my money back – my food bill for the ducks is big enough without having to buy mates for them!

We now had four resident ducks in the Quackery plus any that were just being nursed back to health. My health was still not improving but I had learned to live with it, so people thought I was getting better. No one ever saw me, apart from Vic and Daniel, at the end of the day when I was in so much pain and every muscle in my body felt as though it was on fire. But I was happy and I loved what I was doing. Vic was so understanding and he knew the ducks were my therapy.

On Good Friday we went out for a drive in the car. As I cannot drive far myself, I find I only go to local places. So when we get the chance, Vic likes to take me on longer journeys. On this particular day we went to Busbridge Lakes, Godalming in Surrey, an area I know and like because I was born in Farnham which is close by.

I had no idea where we were going, but Vic knew. He was taking me to a place where many different types of wildfowl are bred. I had often said I liked the pure white Call ducks as they have such pretty faces and they chatter all day long. Vic had made sure that my wheelchair was in the boot of the car because the place we were going covered a vast area.

I could have stayed there all day – they had so many types of birds and as it was the spring time, most of them had their young. Vic took me round the grounds in the wheelchair and then we stopped for some lunch. Afterwards, we went to the gift shop, which was on the site and met the lady who worked there; she was married to the manager of Busbridge Lakes, which is a private wildfowl centre.

I had a long chat with her and told her all about my ducks. She showed me an incubator that had about ten one-day-old white Call ducklings in it. They are not white until they get their feathers – they are pure yellow and just like pictures of ducklings you find in children's books.

Vic asked the manager if they were for sale, but they weren't as they were too young. I told him about all the ducks that I had reared and that I had my own incubator, so he agreed to sell us a pair. He put them into a small box and said they would be fine

61

for the journey home. Vic knows I am always on a diet, so he said these ducklings were instead of an Easter egg. They were beautiful and I chatted to them as we drove home.

We had only been going a little way when we had a heavy storm. It had been sunny all day, but now we had rain followed by a really bad hail storm so that the ground looked as though it was covered in snow. Not bad for April. The fields were white and so were the hedges. So I decided to call the ducks 'Snow' and 'Flake'.

We called in to see my sister, Carol, on the way home and I showed her my Easter present. Carol and her husband Dave have a dog called Jake who's a real softie. I was sitting down with the little box on my lap and Jake came up to it and had a sniff. The ducklings started to chirp and Jake shot behind Carol's chair in surprise. He felt a bit stupid, so came out and had another sniff. Again they chirped, but Jake just sat there with his head going from one side to the other. He had never heard a chirping box before. I placed the box on the floor by my feet and waited to see what Jake would do. He lay down by the box with his head on his paws and as the ducklings chirped, Jake would whimper back. This went on for a long time until Jake realised the box wasn't going to get up and play with him, so he went and found his bone and took it outside to chew.

Snow, the boy, and Flake settled in the incubator when we arrived home and seemed very contented. When they were a couple of days old I let them run around the house, they were so friendly. Like Biscuit, they sat on my feet and nibbled my toes. In the evening they would go to sleep on my lap, or on my shoulder and chew my earrings. The Call duck is a friendlier duck than the mallard and will come up to you and chat away.

When they were old enough to go into the Quackery they decided that they were going to rule the roost. None of the others argued, and Snow and Flake have become good friends of Little Nell and Tootsie, maybe because they are Call ducks too. When Snow was old enough, he knew instinctively what mating was all about and he practised daily. Then he started on Little Nell. I had been told she might not like it because she was blind but this was definitely not the case and she soon developed the habit of going into the pond and calling for Snow. I intend to let them breed and it will be interesting to see if Little Nell wants to incubate her eggs and become a mummy.

Chapter Thirteen

The summer started off rather wet, so I knew we wouldn't have a hose ban that year. However by June it began to get very warm and each day the sun seemed to get hotter and hotter. I used to be a sun worshipper before my illness, but now the heat drains what little energy I have. The ducks were grateful for the shrubs I had planted as they gave them shelter.

The midday sun would shine down on the duck pond, so I would put the garden parasol up over the water to cool it and leave the hose on so that fresh water was constantly trickling into the pond. I know the ducks appreciated this because they would play with the hose and try and catch the water as it came out.

One evening in June, I had a telephone call from Dave at the Wildlife Rescue who had been called out to a major roadworks on the A27 at Patching. There is a pond alongside the road and a female mallard had decided she was not going to nest where all other ducks and swans nest, but had gone across the main road to nest amongst the trees where it was quiet.

What the mallard had not known was, major roadworks were going to take place and a bypass was going to go straight through the area of trees where her nest was. Men had come along and cut down most trees, then the bulldozers had arrived and started to clear the area. When one of these machines starts working, nothing is safe in its path. They had been working for a few weeks and the site was changing daily – they certainly can shift earth when they get going.

It was on one of the very hot days that a workman had

decided to take a break and go and get a cold drink from his van. He was walking past one of the bulldozers and wiping the sweat off his brow with a grubby piece of rag when the sunshine caught something a few feet in front of him. He put his hands up to the driver of the bulldozer to stop him. Luckily, he managed to stop in time, because only about eight feet in front of the machine was the mother duck sitting on her nest. She had no intention of moving – after all, she had a family to hatch, so those men would have to wait.

I'm afraid the Ministry of Transport wouldn't have understood, and the needs of a duck are not important when a road has to be built by a certain time. But the workman who found her had a kind heart and he went and fetched the boss. He parked his van in front of the nest and then fetched some cones and placed them around the back of the nest. She was then safe until they could find out what to do. It is nice to know that the cones do have their good uses, other than littering the countryside.

The boss telephoned the police and told them of their predicament and the police officer gave them the number of Wildlife Rescue. Dave and Sheila went to the work site where the mallard was still sitting on her eggs. As Dave tried to lift the duck up off the nest, to see how many eggs she had got, she flew away. There were twelve eggs in the nest and as Dave picked them up and put them in a box, he knew the mother would not come back. They do not like humans touching their eggs and will desert the nest if they know humans have interfered.

Dave thanked the kind workmen and let them get on with their job. He brought the eggs round to me and I put them in the incubator. It was about two hours since the mother had sat on the eggs, but Dave had kept them warm with a blanket. We had no idea how many days she had been sitting on them, so I waited until it was dark so I could 'candle' them. All twelve were alive and I tried to work out, by the size of the embryos, how many days would pass before they would hatch. By my reckoning, they had nineteen days to go.

Right on time, they started to hatch and by the end of that day, I was a mum to all twelve ducklings. It was the first time I had had all the eggs hatch, so I gave myself a pat on the back. These little ducklings turned out to be pure mallards and I couldn't tell one from the other, so I named them 'The Patching Pack'. I cared for them indoors for the first week, but then put them in the garden as it was so hot. I had to make sure that they kept in the shade because ducklings can get sunstroke.

Vic had been to do some electrical work for an infant school a few days before the eggs hatched and he was telling the headteacher about them. She was very interested and asked if it was possible to bring some of them into school to show the little children. When they had all hatched I phoned the teacher and made arrangements to take them the next day. If children want to handle ducklings it is best if they do it while they are very young. I placed all twelve in a box with a hot water bottle and my faithful old cardigan and they all cuddled up and went to sleep. I asked Daniel to come with me to give me a hand as the thought of thirty little children around frightened the life out of me. My boys were teenagers and older so I had lost touch with the younger generation.

We arrived at the school and were shown into the first classroom. Thirty pairs of beady eyes looked up in anticipation and the teacher told them all to be very quiet and not to make a sudden noise as the lady with the box had something special to show them. You could have heard a pin drop; it was lovely.

I placed the box down very carefully and as I started to lift the lid the twelve ducklings woke up, making a noise that startled the children and their mouths dropped open in surprise. The teacher had made the children sit on the floor in a big circle and as I put the ducklings down, all twelve of them ran in different directions. There were squeals of delight which frightened the babies so I put them back in the box and then took out one at a time so the children could hold or stroke them.

We then went on to the next class where I just passed one duckling around at a time for the children to hold. This proved a lot easier on my nerves and better for the ducklings' well-being. In each class we visited the children were progressively older, so they asked sensible questions, except one little boy. I think he had just been told off by his teacher before Daniel and I arrived as he had a very sullen face. When I asked him if he had any questions for me, he asked, 'Do they mess themselves a lot and does it smell?' What a nice little boy!

It took us nearly an hour to go round all the classrooms.

When we had finished the ducklings were very tired, I was shattered, and even Daniel was tired. I think it was the result of all the questions being asked all at the same time – if you didn't answer them straightaway, the children would talk louder and louder.

The Patching Pack recovered from their school experience and grew into fine ducks, but I often wonder what would have happened if there hadn't been any roadworks and the mother mallard had hatched her own brood. Ducklings must get food and water within twenty-four hours of hatching and since the only water near the nest was on the other side of the A27, in the pond, she would have had to walk her babies across the busy main road without getting them run over. Somehow I don't think she would have made it. If you ever see a duck walking across a road with her family behind her, just remember the Patching Pack, and how they nearly didn't make it. Also, be patient and give the ducks time to cross, because if they have only recently hatched, they will be very tired and hungry.

Chapter Fourteen

The heat wave continued and I was finding the weather very tiring. Other M.E. sufferers were struggling as well. Although it was lovely to have such fine weather, I was not well enough to appreciate it. I spent a lot of the day sleeping, and then did my chores during the evening, but when it was bed time I couldn't sleep. Some nights I would just go outside and sit on my favourite top step and watch the wildlife. They seem to talk to each other even though they appear to be asleep. The moon would shine down on Widewater and I often thought we had two moons. The reflection was perfect, and sometimes the swans would sit on the reflection and clean themselves.

Another reason I like the early hours of the morning is because you can watch your world waking up. The process starts when the ducks and swans have a quick clean up, putting their feathers back in the right places. Then they all take turns in lifting their bodies slightly out of the water before stretching their necks as far as they can and flapping their wings so hard, that every part of their bodies is brought back to life. Then the starlings and sparrows begin to wake up and start their dawn chorus. Once all the wildlife has started to stir, the sun begins to rise and then the birds are safe to start hunting for food. Each morning is so different from the next and the clouds can change the scene every few seconds. Some days the sun is so bright you think it will burn itself out before the rest of the world is awake.

While Vic and Daniel are still in the land of nod, the wildlife are busy with their day. Once the birds have had their wash and brush up they come into the garden. They always wait

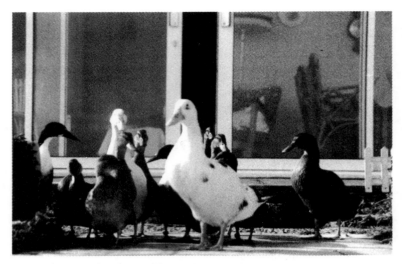
'Come on, Mum, where is our breakfast?'

until the light is good because we have cats that live in the neighbourhood who insist on teasing the ducks. I am getting quite good at throwing handfuls of soil at the cats, but they are now wise to me and they have learned to duck (excuse the pun).

There are at least seventy ducks who come to me for their breakfast. The ones that I have reared come right up to me and follow me into the shed where the corn is kept. The visitors stay in the water, but come as close to the garden as possible and wait for breakfast. I then fill a black bucket with the food and start to throw the corn all over the ground. It is a most satisfying feeling, knowing these birds are here because they want to be – they are free to fly away but they don't. They trust me and that makes me feel wonderful. I know there are people who are perfectly healthy, and wealthy, but have never had such a rich closeness with nature as I have and I know that if I hadn't got this awful illness, I might not have known such happiness.

Chapter Fifteen

My friends at Wildlife Rescue told me that at the end of August there is an open day for the local wildlife hospital. I had never been there before and Vic said it would be a good idea to go, but I don't think he realised what he was letting himself in for.

We arrived at Brent Lodge Hospital near Chichester and the entrance fee was either tins of dog food or a donation. I liked their sense of humour! We drove in and all along the driveway were large fenced-in areas containing swans, seagulls, cormorants and herons. They were all recovering from some injury or other. I noticed how content they all were, and I knew I was going to like this place.

We parked in the car park and were greeted by an enormous long-haired Alsatian. He was very friendly and I gave him a pat on his head. As we couldn't see anybody around (it had only been open for ten minutes), I asked the dog if he was in charge. He never replied, but turned and started to walk towards a door. Then out came a gentleman who happened to be the owner, but I think his dog thought he was the boss and the man was his understudy. He welcomed us with a big smile and asked us if we had been there before. We explained it was our first visit, so he gave us a map of the area. This was just as well as the hospital covered a wide area. We decided to start at the hospital itself and then work around to where the birds convalesced. There were signposts to the entrance of the hospital and as we opened the door a voice shouted, 'Go away'. It sounded as if the staff weren't too friendly.

I should have realised that as you walk into the hospital, you are greeted by Charlie the parrot. He did look funny – he had a beautiful crest of feathers on his head and a lovely red, blue and green back. But there were no feathers on his chest at all and on the front he was as bald as a coot. Apparently, his owner neglected him and he got bored, so he had decided to pluck himself. He enjoyed it so much that even though he was now living at the hospital, he still continued to pluck. I said to the 'carer' that he might grow out of it now that he was living there and there was a lot going on to keep him amused, but he explained they had had him for seven years and he still plucked himself.

The hospital ward was very well set out: there were cages of all sizes, all around, sometimes as many as four on top of each other. Nearly all of them were occupied by a different creature or bird. There were hedgehogs, squirrels and birds, all in clean warm containers with a card clipped to the outside of each cage. On the card was the type of creature, its sex, where it was found, what was wrong with it and details of its treatment. So there was no chance of getting the wrong card with the wrong bird and it seemed to us to be a very good system.

There were quite a few carers helping out as volunteers and everyone seemed very happy. They were a lovely group of people and were very keen to answer any questions – they certainly knew their job. Vic and I spent at least an hour in the hospital and could have stayed there longer but it was becoming very crowded. We never realised it would be so popular, but now we have been there we know what the attraction is. I had noticed that one of the cages contained a male mallard which had been shot with an air rifle. It had lost one eye and the other was badly injured. I asked one of the helpers what would happen to him and he said he wasn't sure, but would go and see the warden in charge.

The warden was a lovely lady called Penny, and she spent a long time talking to us about what goes on in the hospital. I could have listened to her for hours as she really knew her job and loved it. I explained about our interest in wildlife and about the Quackery and said that if we could help with convalescence she should let me know. She said that once they had done all they could for the duck, they would have to have somewhere where the duck could live his last days in safety. As a result, he came and lived with us. He is known as Nelson and like Little Nell, he soon found his way around the garden.

After we had finished in the hospital, we looked around the grounds and saw all the birds that were now getting their strength back ready to be released again back to where they were found. I was surprised at the different breeds of birds that they had – buzzards, owls, jays, rooks, crows, plus the coastal birds we were used to. Considering that this hospital is run solely on charity, it does not skimp on anything. The cages are spotless and there is plenty of food for the inmates. The organisation is dedicated to caring for wildlife and if it weren't for my illness, I would not hesitate in going to work for it.

About a month after going to Brent Lodge, I had a phone call from Penny. She had a female mallard that was born with a deformed leg. It was quite capable of surviving in the wild, because the duck used the bad leg as a balance, so she would hop everywhere. Penny had released her back onto the pond where she was found, but members of the public had brought her back to the hospital four times, because they thought she had a broken leg. So Penny asked me if I would have her. She apologised for giving me another mouth to feed and said she didn't get many ducks that couldn't be set free again; this one should be the last for that year.

On the way home from the hospital I was chatting to the duck and asking her what she would like to be called. I couldn't call her Hoppirty because we have a seagull with a bad leg and he has that name. So I asked her if she would like to be called Penelope, after the warden and she quacked at me in agreement. Penelope soon settled in with the others in the Quackery and she can hop to the top of the garden as fast as the two-legged ducks.

Only three days later that I had another phone call from Penny. She wasn't sure how I would react and hesitated a bit so I had to tell her to 'spit it out'. Her latest victim was a male mallard that had been picked up the day I collected Penelope. He was in such a bad state that they had thought he would die within an hour or two, so they left him quietly in a box and waited. He was still alive later that day so Penny and the vet examined him. He had no tail and no feathers on his back and hardly any on his wings; he was bleeding and he must have been badly attacked. But what was worse was his beak: the top of the beak looked as though it had been hit by a car and the bill had been pushed back on itself, so it was only three-quarters of its original length. When he had his beak closed it looked as though the lower bill was a spoon. They cleaned up his wounds and gave him an injection of antibiotics to stop any germs making him worse then left him to recover from his ordeal. Goodness knows what he had been through and they were surprised when, two days later, he was trying to clean himself.

So Penny asked me if I would take him on and nurse him back to health. I was only too pleased to help but I was feeling very tired and I couldn't drive far that day. She said there was no hurry as she understood my illness – a friend of hers had got M.E. so she knew how its victims could feel poorly on one day and pretty good on another.

The next day I went back to the hospital and saw Penny about the duck. She was very excited because the duck was trying to eat, which could only be a good sign. We walked into the ward and I was greeted with 'Go away'. 'Good morning, Charlie,' I said and gave him a stroke on his bald front – it was as if he had a permanent five o'clock shadow on his chest. He spent his day on top of the cage and loved any amount of attention anyone would give him. I asked Penny if he would ever be re-housed, but she said they had all grown very fond of him and couldn't let him go.

We went to the far side of the ward where the duck was resting. Penny turned to me and with a very serious look on her face she said, 'Now promise me you are not going to laugh when I get him out.' What on earth was I about to see?

Penny turned away to get the duck and when she turned back she was trying very hard not to smile. The poor little duck looked so funny – he was nearly bald and his beak looked as though he was smiling all the time. They thought he had been hit by a car and then the other ducks had tried to kill him (they do that if a bird is badly injured as it saves him or her from suffering too much). Penny said that if I didn't want to take him on, then she would have him put to sleep. It would take up too much time to nurse him back to health but they knew I had the time and the place and that I was mad about ducks. I put the duck in my pet carrier and was ready to go home, when I remembered to tell her that I had named the last duck after her. She was really pleased and honoured. 'What are you going to call that one?' she asked, pointing at the carrier. I said he was like a cartoon character that had gone wrong and I would have to think of a name, but what?

On the way home I chatted to the duck and was thinking of different names I could give him, but none seemed to fit, so I decided to wait and ask Vic. I put the duck in the Quackery and Snow went up to him and bit him on the side. That was the only time any of the ducks hurt him and I think it was Snow's way of telling him that he was in charge. He never did it to any of the females but I think he was following a law of the wild that they have.

I made myself a cup of tea and went and sat on my top step to watch the new duck. He must have felt very embarrassed about his looks because he went and hid in one of the hutches for a while. When he had plucked up enough courage, he came out and went and had a drink of water. He managed that without any trouble, then he went over to the bowl of corn. The duck was having difficulty getting the food up, so I filled the bowl up so that he could put his beak in deeper and fill the lower bill with corn. Then he lifted his head up and seemed to flick the food along the bottom bill before opening the top one to grab the food before it fell on the ground. This worked well and he spent a long time filling his tummy as he must have been really hungry.

That evening when Vic came home from work I introduced him to the new duck. Vic couldn't help but smile, the duck looked so comical. When anyone saw him, they smiled, and we therefore decided to call him 'Smiler'. Each day Smiler improved his eating method and soon he had it off to a fine art. My only worry was the state of his feathers, so Vic took some photos of him, so that we would be able to judge whether they were improving.

We need not have worried. Four months after Smiler came to live with us, we saw a great improvement. He now has all his feathers and even a tail and the only way of telling him apart from all the other drakes is that he always looks happy because he's always smiling.

Chapter Sixteen

The same year that Smiler came to live with us a neighbour phoned us to say that a very young seagull was at the bottom of her garden. She said it looked as though it was soaked – all its feathers were hanging down and water was dripping off them. I knew at once that this meant the seagull was not waterproof and either it had been hand-reared and escaped, or it was ill.

Vic and I went along to the house and took the pet-carrier with us. We knew that seagulls could be quite vicious, so Vic took some thick gardening gloves to protect his hands. The poor seagull looked like a drowned rat. He was standing on a large stone and I could see he was shivering. Gently, Vic bent down and lifted the bird up and I helped put it in the carrier. We thanked the lady and said we would let her know how we got on.

As soon as we arrived back home I telephoned Dave to ask his advice. He said he would call round later and meanwhile we were to keep the gull in the Quackery until he had dried off. Thank goodness it was a lovely hot day. The gull seemed to accept me being in the garden and when I offered him bread, he walked up, slowly at first, then he took the food from me as though he hadn't eaten for ages. Once he had filled his tummy, he set to and cleaned up his feathers. The ducks didn't bother him so I left them to do their own thing and went and got on with a few jobs of my own. Dave turned up a little while later and asked me to fetch the bird (which was a juvenile herring gull) out of the ducks' garden so that he could have a good look at it. He watched me and said that he must have been reared by humans because he was so tame.

After giving the bird a check-up, we both agreed that there was nothing wrong with it, so once he had dried out completely, I could let him go free. I left him with the ducks overnight and next day he looked quite alright, so after feeding all the wildfowl, I let him out and put him on the lawn. That is where he stayed all day – he was not in the least bit interested in the water. Dave had given me some raw fish to feed him and he soon tucked into it as though I hadn't given him anything the night before. A few of the wild seagulls tried to take the fish away from him, but he just shouted at them and hunched up his shoulders to make himself look aggressive.

A whole week had gone by and the gull was still in our garden. He would follow me down to the water's edge when I fed the ducks and then he would fly back up to our house and stand on Whistler's footpath. One day I left the patio doors open as it was such a lovely warm day, and he hopped onto the doorstep and looked in. I was busy in the kitchen and when I walked into the lounge and saw him looking in, it made me jump. 'Oh, hello Fred,' I said. Now that is a good name, I thought, and Fred seemed to agree.

Every morning, Fred would be on the footpath waiting for his breakfast. He would frighten all the other seagulls away by screaming at them, or chasing them as he was never in any mood for sharing his breakfast with anyone. I had used up all the raw fish that Dave had given me, so the next time I went to the supermarket, I bought the shop's own brand of tinned dog food. A large tin lasted two days and at 14p a tin, it was not going to break the bank.

Late one afternoon, I was getting the meal ready for the evening and as I turned to get a plate from the cupboard, I saw Fred standing in the doorway of the kitchen and lounge. 'And what do you want then, Fred?' I asked. He walked into the kitchen and watched me get his tin of dog food from the fridge, then followed me out to the footpath and stood next to me while I filled his dish for him.

Every day, as long as it was dry, I had the patio doors open, so Fred could come in. He would wander into the kitchen and look up at the fridge, willing me to get him his food. One afternoon he settled on the rug by my chair and had a rest with me. Slowly I tamed him enough for him to take the food out of my hand. He was a real character and when it was raining and I had the doors closed, he would tap on the window to be let in, but I made him stay outside.

Gradually, Fred started going into the water for a wash and brush up and he would also have a fly around but he was never gone long. He would circle overhead and scream at the top of his voice, 'Look Mum, I can fly.' He would then land on the shed roof and have a good look round to make sure there were no other gulls around. Then, if it was all clear, he would fly down onto the footpath and wait for his next meal.

In our local evening paper there appeared an article asking people to write in if they had an interesting story to tell. As there is so much sad news nowadays in the papers, I thought the story of Fred might amuse people, so I telephoned the paper and explained about my seagull. The very next day someone phoned back and arranged for the photographer to come. I went and told Fred he was going to be a celebrity so he had a wash and brush up in the small bird bath which we have on one of the steps leading down to the water's edge. I felt like offering him a mirror and comb.

When the photographer arrived complete with camera and spare films, he was so surprised to see the gull waiting on the path. I introduced them to each other and Fred went and sat back on the bird bath and raised his head slightly, as if to say, 'This is my best side.' The man took many pictures and then asked me if the gull would take food from me. I went and got his tin of dog food and started to spoon the food onto the floor. Fred must have known he was to become a star because he started to eat straight from the spoon and all I could hear was the click, click, click of the camera.

About a week later Fred's picture was in the newspaper and I had quite a few phone calls from friends saying they had seen it. I have had a word with Fred and he has agreed that I can be his agent if I want, now that he is a star. He stayed with us all summer and winter, then in the spring he went off to find himself a mate. I am hoping he will bring her here to meet us and if he does, I'll name her Ginger. So I shall have Fred and Ginger to keep me company along with all the ducks and swans, while Vic is at work.

Chapter Seventeen

Over the past few years I have learned so much about wildlife and how to care for the sick or injured. It has helped me cope with my disease and even though I still suffer from myalgic encephalomyelitis, I don't let it rule my life. My husband, sons and ducks need me as much as I need them and I try and keep my spirits up. Some days I just feel too ill so I spend the day in my chair with my feet up and rest as much as possible because I know that tomorrow is another day and I might feel completely different.

However, one major lesson I have learned is that nature knows best. I thought I could do better than nature and I tried to interfere with it once at the expense of a dear little duck called Churchill. It all started one morning when I had a phone call to say a duckling had been found at the back of a factory and it seemed to be very weak. I asked if it was possible to bring the bird to me as my arms and shoulders were hurting and I knew I wouldn't have the strength to steer the car. (I never ever drive when I am feeling so weak.)

The young girl came to my house with the little duckling in a small box. It seemed that a mallard had nested at the back of one of the factories on the Churchill Industrial Estate. The lake was on the other side of the road and that morning the staff had watched the mother duck walk her young family across the road to the water. The girl realised that there were only twelve ducklings in the procession and when she had first found the nest there had been thirteen eggs. Once the ducks were safely across the road, she went to see if the last egg was still there.

Lying in the deserted nest was a very weak and feeble-looking duckling with nothing for company but broken egg shells. I took a good look at the duckling and I could see that it had been attacked. The back of his neck had blood on it, his beak had been bitten and a small piece was missing, and his legs were very wobbly as though he had not yet tried to stand and walk. I thanked the young girl and said I would do what I could for it, but I had my doubts.

I closed the front door and went to find my old cardigan and the hot water bottle. I sat on my chair with the bottle and cardigan on my lap, then placed the little duckling on top, cupping my hands over him to make him feel safe and warm. The heat from the hot water bottle was doing me good as well and I was soon fast asleep.

I only woke up when the duckling started to move about and try and get out from under my hands. I looked at the clock and found we had both been asleep for an hour. I picked up the bird and had a good look at him. He had fluffed up now so he looked a lot better, but his neck didn't look right. I placed him on the floor and he started to walk towards my feet (ducklings have a thing about naked toes). Then I realised why his neck looked odd: I think the mother duck had tried to kill the baby by breaking its neck, but had only dislocated it.

I telephoned Dave and he came over later in the day to see what could be done, if anything, for this poor little unwanted fellow. In the meantime I fed him and he seemed to manage to eat without any difficulty. But when he walked about he seemed to go sideways like a crab. I let him sleep on my chair with the hot water bottle and we waited for Dave to come.

Dave said that the missing piece of beak should grow back and explained that though his legs were weak, he would get better as he recovered his strength. As for his neck, Dave said it was not dislocated because it didn't hurt him when he massaged it; he might have been growing in the egg like that and that might have been why the mother had tried to kill him at birth. It is the survival of the fittest in the wild; a sick weakling would draw attention to itself and put all its brothers and sisters in danger, so the parent tries to kill it as soon as it is born. Though it seems cruel, this course of action makes sense.

When Vic came home from work that night he took one look

at the duckling and said he looked like Quasimodo when he walked on account of his shoulder sticking up which looked like a hump. I didn't like that name so we named him Churchill as that was where he was found.

I was advised to massage the duckling's neck as often as possible while it was still very tiny and maybe it would grow straight. The little duckling enjoyed his daily massage and would lie for hours on my lap while I gently rubbed his neck and tried to push it back to the right position. Each day he became stronger and would run around the house like a crab, always going sideways. It wasn't long before he could walk over to his food and water in a straight line, sideways, which was a very funny sight. Dave called round most days to see how the duck was doing and as he was not in any pain, Dave thought he would just be an odd duck but live a full and happy life. We would have to wait to see if he would ever be able to fly.

In the evenings the duckling would be asleep on my lap or he would climb up onto my shoulder and tuck his head under my hair. He was a very friendly little bird and I would let him follow me around the house or sit with me in the garden. He was never very far away from me and when I needed my sleep, he would have his at the same time and lie outstretched on my lap. I became very fond of Churchill as I could relate to his problem. His neck muscle seemed to be very weak and when I held his head and pulled gently, his neck would go straight, but as soon as I let go it would go back into an 'S' shape and along his body, so that his head was by his left wing.

It was amazing to watch him wash himself. He had no problem doing his left side, but when he needed to clean down his right-hand side, he would lean against the chair or wall and swing his head right around and clean himself quickly before his head would swing back to the left, as though it was on a very strong spring. I sometimes need to wear a neck collar because I have problems with my muscles and I wondered if one could be made for Churchill. However, this was not advisable as the collar would stop him from eating or cleaning and as ducks grow so fast, we would have had to keep making the collar bigger each day.

When Churchill was four weeks old I took him out into the Quackery to meet the other residents. They took no notice of him and carried on worm-hunting. I had wondered if they would pick on him because he was deformed, but no, eating was more important. Churchill joined in the worm-hunt and I sat and watched him from my favourite top step. He soon found the pond and after examining the edges he decided he would have a go at swimming. That was a lovely sight as he had no problem and could swim and dive and splash like any other duck.

Churchill moved into the Quackery that night and he slept with Little Nell and Tootsie. Each day he seemed stronger but his neck looked more deformed as he grew. When he was six weeks old, his feathers started to grow and I noticed that the weight of each feather on his little wings was too much for him and they would drag on the floor. Also, his neck was becoming weaker and he wasn't walking around much. It was easier for him to simply lie down with his neck on the floor, just like dogs do when they are hot and tired.

I asked Dave to come and see him again and after giving the duckling a thorough check over he said that he believed the duck had a muscle problem. As he grew more feathers, he would become weaker. He suggested taping up the wings for a few days to see if that would help (that is what they do if a bird has a broken wing). Churchill didn't seem to mind having his wings bound up and I think it was better for him. But his neck become weaker and he now couldn't hold his head up long enough to feed himself.

Dave, Sheila and I talked it over the next week and we all said it was cruel keeping little Churchill alive as he was getting weaker. So Dave took him home and humanely put my little duck to sleep.

That night I cried, not because I had lost a lovely duck, but because he had something wrong with him that was so like my own illness. He had very weak muscles and the only kind thing we could do for him was to end his life. His mother had known right at the start that there was something wrong with her baby, so that is why she had wanted to put him out of his misery. Then I had come along and had thought I knew better; I had tried to keep him alive, but he had only got worse.

I do hope Churchill understood that I had acted for what I thought was his own sake, not because I thought I could do better than nature and prolong his life for my own satisfaction.

Nature has been doing her job a lot longer than I have, and I have learned that my job is to help the birds that can have a good quality of life and leave her to do what is right for those little ones that are too poorly to live.

I am very grateful for one thing: I am not a duckling with M.E. or I would not he here and you would not be reading this book.

Chapter Eighteen

My interest in ducks had begun to rub off on Vic and he would take me to the wildlife reserves at the weekends to learn as much as we could about ducks and their environment. It was very satisfying to know that we were doing a good job and that our ducks were happy and contented in the reserve. Even at the time of writing, we are still learning and there are always new things to find out. It is this which makes ducks such an interesting hobby.

On one of our visits to a local reserve, there was a demonstration of wood carving. The craftsmen were carving the most wonderful birds – wrens, owls, eagles and, you guessed it, ducks. It was just as well that I was in my wheelchair because we were watching the carvers for such a long time. I couldn't move away and time just seemed to stand still.

Vic started to talk to a gentleman who was carving a mallard and it was awe-inspiring. Neither of us had seen such magnificent carvings and we couldn't leave without finding out more about this skill. Vic had so many questions to ask. I knew what was going through his mind – he is very good with his hands and it shows in the DIY jobs that he's done around the home. He is never satisfied unless he has done his best and the more I looked at the carvings, the more I knew Vic could do them and do them well. We spent more than two hours talking to the carvers and Vic was told that there was a new course starting in the autumn. We took all the details and later Vic applied to go on the course.

Vic thoroughly enjoyed himself on the two-day course.

When he came home with his finished product – a magnificent carving of a golden-eye duck – I was amazed how quickly he had picked up the skill. He was so pleased with himself that I knew he had found a hobby that he would enjoy.

So now we have live ducks in the garden and carved ducks indoors. Vic has carved a plover, a mallard and a red-breasted merganser to go with the golden-eye and he is about to start a duck in flight. It is lovely to be able to share a hobby like ours, especially now the children have grown up and have lives of their own, so that we feel we can do things for ourselves and not feel guilty.

At the weekends I am to be found sitting on the top step watching the ducks who will be swimming, cleaning their feathers or just resting on the water. Vic will have a lump of wood on his lap, whittling away for hours. It sounds as if we are Darby and Joan in the making, but it is so relaxing and it does me the world of good.

Vic found he had another talent we didn't know about when I brought home a gardening magazine containing an article on how to do topiary (the art of training and cutting trees and shrubs into shapes). At the top end of the Quackery there is a small, low privet hedge, so Vic decided that would be where he would have a go at doing topiary. It's a hobby which needs a lot of patience because the shapes take all season to grow. But now we have a duck growing out of the hedge, it is a talking point when people see it. As I name all my ducks, I felt this one needed a name as well, but what could I call him? It took us a while to decide, then we both agreed on the name: 'D.For', that is, D for duck.

It is now seven years since I was diagnosed as having M.E. and it took me a couple of years to accept it. I joined two organisations that help people with this illness, the M.E. Association and Action for M.E. and they have proved to be my lifelines. There have been some very bad days when I have not been able to face the future, but these organisations have been there to help – all I had to do was phone them. Also, we have a local group of sufferers and carers and we support each other, keeping in touch between meetings by way of a newsletter of which I was editor for three years, till I found it was draining my energy.

A few months ago I woke up one morning and found I hadn't got a voice. I just couldn't speak and when I tried, my voice was like a sore whisper, but my throat was not sore. I didn't know if this was yet another symptom of M.E. so when I went to see my doctor I asked him. He had not heard of anyone with this problem but said it might get better on its own, because when he looked in my mouth there was neither inflammation nor spots.

A month later the condition, far from getting better, had grown worse. After saying good morning to Vic, the voice started to fade away. By the time he set off for work there was no sound coming from my throat. I started to panic, so phoned the M.E. helpline to find out if they knew if it might be something to do with the M.E. They couldn't say for sure so suggested that I should ask my doctor to send me to a specialist. This he did and I received an appointment within two weeks.

The hospital was very good and the specialist said that there was no cancer (which was a relief) nor any growths on my voice-box. This had simply stopped working and the doctor thought it was quite likely to be on account of the illness as the voice-box is a muscle and my muscles don't work properly anymore. The specialist made an appointment for me to go to a speech therapist to see if that would help. I had to wait only five days to see her. She was a lovely person and gave me breathing exercises to do. However, these had to be discontinued because they made me feel weak and ill. The therapist realised that any form of exercise would make me ill and she said she believed the M.E. was the cause of my loss of voice. I was to learn sign language and rest my voice as much as possible. Sign language is all very well in front of people, but I still cannot master it on the telephone.

We heard many comments on how nice it must be for Vic not having me talking, but after a while it became very frustrating. It was sixteen weeks before I recovered my voice and I still dread getting a cold or sore throat in case it goes again. My family and my doctor have been most supportive – they try to understand what the illness is doing to me and they are there when I need them. Our youngest son, Daniel, was living at home when I became ill and he has been very helpful. Whenever I have felt too ill to look after the ducks, he has done it for me. He has also become a dab hand at making me cups of tea (by now it must be apparent that I'm a tea-aholic).

The ducks have kept me sane during my illness. They seem to know when I'm feeling really down because they keep chatting to me as though they are saying 'We need you, Mum.' That lovely little duck called Plucky will never know how grateful I am to him – he may have lived only three days, but he has left his mark on my life and I thank him.

The Quackery and all who live in it have given me hours of pleasure. There was Snow and Flake, Little Nell and her sister Tootsie (she has never forgiven me for giving her that medicine). Then we have Penelope and Nelson; the tufty ducks, Bright Eyes and Tufty, and, last of all, Smiler. I thank them all for their trust in me and the love they have shown.

I often think of Blondie and Whistler and their three little babies and I'm quite convinced that they are on duty by the Pearly Gates. I do hope they have met up with Biscuit and that they can all walk that footpath together. But most of all, I would like to thank the man who has been by my side through thick and thin and who has been so supportive where the ducks are concerned. We have laughed and cried about some of them, but we have done it together and that has meant so much to me. He has encouraged me because he has seen how much help the birds have been to me through my illness. They have helped me to forget about my pain and have shown me so much trust.

Most important of all, my husband has always been by my side, helping me and listening to me, even when I have moaned. He has seen me in pain and has known when to fuss over me and when to leave me alone. Vic cheers me up on my bad days and enjoys and shares the good days; sometimes he has let me do things even if it has made me more ill. I have had to learn my own limitations. He is a wonderful man, I love him dearly and I am so glad we have shared the lovely world of ducks.

So thank you Vic from ME AND MY DUCKS.